Herbs for a Healthy Pregnancy

Penelope Ody majored in chemistry at Bristol University in England. Later, she studied herbal medicine at the School of Phytotherapy in Sussex and traditional Chinese medicine at the College of Traditional Chinese Medicine in Guangzhou. She is a member of the National Institute of Medical Herbalists, England's leading professional body for practicing herbalists. Ody's previous herb books include *The Complete Medicinal Herbal*, *Home Herbal*, *Handbook of Over-the-Counter Herbal Medicines*, *Pocket Medicinal Herbs*, *101 Great Natural Remedies*, and *Herbs for First Aid*.

Ody's herb garden in Buckinghamshire, where she practiced as a consultant medical herbalist for ten years, has been featured on BBC Television. She now lives in Hampshire and continues to contribute to a number of publications worldwide and to lecture on herbal medicine around the globe.

Herbs for a Healthy Pregnancy

Penelope Ody

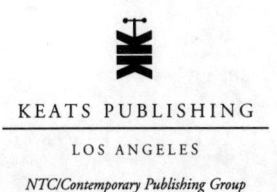

KEATS PUBLISHING
LOS ANGELES
NTC/Contemporary Publishing Group

Herbs for a Healthy Pregnancy is intended solely for educational and informational purposes and not as medical advice. Please consult a medical or health professional if you have an questions about your health.

Library of Congress Cataloging-in-Publication Data

Ody, Penelope.
    Herbs for a healthy pregnancy/ from conception to childbirth / Penelope Ody.
           p.   cm.
    Includes bibliographical references and index.
    ISBN 0-87983-986-4 (paper)
    1. Herbs—Therapeutic use. 2. Pregnancy. I.Title.
RM666.H33013817   1999
615'.321—dc21   99-33156
                                                                  CIP

Published by Keats Publishing.
A division of NTC/Contemporary Publishing Group, Inc.
4255 West Touhy Avenue, Lincolnwood, Illinois 60646-1975 U.S.A.

Copyright © 1999 by Penelope Ody.

All rights reserved. No part of this work may be reproduced, stored in a retrieval system, or transmitted in any form or by any means electronic, mechanical, photocopying, recording, or otherwise, without the prior permission of NTC/Contemporary Publishing Group, Inc.

Printed in the United States of America

International Standard Book Number: 0-87983-986-4

99 00 01 02 03 04 RRD 18 17 16 15 14 13 12 11 10 9 8 7 6 5 4 3 2 1

*For mothers everywhere
but especially for mine, Mary Hebron Ody,
and for hers, my grandmother,
Mary Hannah Tweddell (1879–1963)*

Contents

Introduction	xi
1. PLANNING FOR CHILDBIRTH	1
Preconception and Conception	2
Dealing with Infertility	5
2. PREGNANCY	9
Monthly Progress: The Fetus	9
Monthly Progress: The Mother	11
Diet	14
Exercise	18
Massage	21
3. EASING THE DISCOMFORTS OF PREGNANCY	23
Abdominal Pain	23
Allergies	24
Iron-Deficiency Anemia	25
Backache	27
Bladder and Kidney Problems	28
Breathlessness	29
Carpal Tunnel Syndrome	29
Constipation	30
Edema (Fluid Retention)	31
Fainting and Low Blood Pressure	32
Fatigue and Emotional Upsets	33
Heartburn	34
Hemorrhoids	35
Hiatal Hernia	36

Insomnia	36
Leg Cramps	37
Morning Sickness	38
Sinusitus	40
Stress	41
Stretch Marks	42
Teeth and Gum Problems	44
Vaginal Yeast Infection	44
Varicose Veins	45
4. MORE SERIOUS CONDITIONS OF PREGNANCY	**47**
Ectopic Pregnancy	47
High Blood Pressure	48
Preeclampsia	49
Symphysis Pubis Dysfunction (SPD)	50
Threatened Miscarriage	51
5. CHILDBIRTH	**53**
Preparing for Childbirth	53
Breech Babies	54
During Labor	55
Herbal Birthing Kit	58
6. AFTER THE BIRTH	**61**
Afterpains	62
Contraction of the Uterus	62
Perineum Problems	62
Postnatal Depression	63
The Shock of Parenthood	64
Tiredness	65
Stillbirth	66
7. BREAST-FEEDING	**67**
Preparing for Breast-Feeding	67
Engorgement	69

Insufficient Milk	69
Mastitis	70
Sore and Cracked Nipples	71

8. EASING BABY'S DISCOMFORTS WITH HERBS ... 73
    - Colds — 73
    - Colic — 74
    - Cradle Cap — 75
    - Diaper Rash — 76
    - Eye Problems — 76
    - Jaundice — 77
    - Sleeplessness — 78
    - Teething — 79
    - Umbilical Care — 79
    - Yeast Infection — 80

9. HERBS TO AVOID DURING PREGNANCY ... 81

10. *Materia Medica* ... 91

11. HOW TO PREPARE HERBAL REMEDIES
    - Infusions — 143
    - Decoctions — 144
    - Combined Infusions and Decoctions — 144
    - Infused Oils — 145
    - Massage Oils — 145
    - Compresses — 146
    - Poultices — 146
    - Tinctures — 146
    - Buying and Storing Herbs — 148

Herb Suppliers ... 149
Glossary ... 151
References ... 157
Index ... 159

Introduction

Modern pregnancy and childbirth, with their emphasis on clinical intervention and electronic monitoring, are far removed from the world of our grandmothers and great-grandmothers—where births took place at home with the support of only friends and relatives and with a few suitable herbs to help. Given the high mortality rate for both mothers and babies in those days, no one would want a return to such basic techniques.

Many would agree, however, that the current popularity of Caesarean sections and inducing labor so that baby's arrival will match the hospital timetable have veered a little too far in the direction of invasive medicine. In addition, the political correctness of avoiding every food or beverage that carries even the remotest risk of crossing the placental barrier verges, at times, on the neurotic.

Somewhere in between, no doubt, lies the correct balance, where traditional remedies and homespun wisdom sit side by side with today's high-tech medicine to achieve a healthy and holistic pregnancy—creating physical, emotional, and spiritual well-being, with a relaxed and happy mother and a happy, healthy baby as well.

Herbs can play a part in this vision by helping to ease the minor ills of pregnancy, to soothe the pains of childbirth, and to set baby on the road to a contented and well-balanced life. Herbs have a long tradition of such use, as their very names remind us: motherwort was used to calm anxieties and tension during the birth, mother's hearts (better known as shepherd's purse) to heal postpartum bleeding, and lady's mantle to strengthen the womb and ready it for labor. Traditional herb country names are often a good indication of their original use. In Europe, you often find "mother's" or "lady's" in the names of such herbs, while among Native Americans "squaw" in herbs' names is a similar pointer to gynecological action.

Native Americans, such as the Menominees, used the leaves of partridge berry (*Mitchella repens*)—also known as squaw vine or squaw plum—to ease labor pains. Various species of *Trillium*, generally known as birthroot or squaw flower, were used by the tribes around Lake Superior in the same way. The roots of the white-flowered *Trillium grandiflorum* (also called squaw flower and now a popular shade plant for garden borders) were used by the Potawatomis to soothe sore nipples during breast-feeding.

Many of these herbs were also used as abortifacients on both sides of the Atlantic. European pennyroyal (*Mentha pulegium*)—a dangerous herb that is more likely to cause fetal damage than an abortion—has its New World equivalent in American pennyroyal or squaw mint (*Hedeoma pulegioides*), which was recommended by the early settlers for "obstructed menses" and certainly leads to abortion in cattle. Liferoot (*Senecio aureus*), which was used by the Catawbas to ease childbirth pains and hasten delivery, was also known as squaw weed; taken at other times in the pregnancy, it too can damage the fetus.

For centuries, women had a monopoly on midwifery, using the herbs and charms their mothers and grandmothers had taught them. In the Middle Ages, many of these traditions—which no doubt date back to pagan times—were fiercely criticized by the church, and many midwives were condemned as witches and burnt at the stake. After birth, babies had to be taken to the local priest to be examined for signs of bewitchment, and the church went to great lengths to instruct midwives in the correct form of baptism so the weak and stillborn could be given the appropriate Christian blessing to speed them to heaven. In many areas of sixteenth-century England, midwives, in addition to having their skills monitored by physicians, were regularly examined by the local bishop to ensure that they were not in league with the devil and had no plans to sell the souls of their newborn charges. Many of these attitudes arrived in North America with the European settlers, leading to subsequent witch-hunts in New England.

By the seventeenth century, male midwives were becoming more commonplace, a phenomenon of which herbalist Nicholas Culpeper (1616–1653) heartily disapproved. He urged traditional women healers to study his herbal writings. "If you make use of them," he wrote, "you will find your work easier, you will need not call for help of a Man-Midwife, which is a disparagement, not only to yourselves, but also to your Professions. All the Perfections that can be in a woman, ought to be in a Midwife . . ."

At a time when childbirth was a major cause of female mortality, skilled midwives were much in demand and were rewarded accordingly. Not surprisingly, the predominantly male physicians of the eighteenth century tried to take over this lucrative profession. Until well into the 1700s, many women were recorded as notable obstetricians, gynecologists, and general physicians; however, as the medical profession became more codified and formalized in the nineteenth century, women in Europe—and to a lesser extent in the United States—were barred from the recognized medical schools, and male physicians began to assume roles that had traditionally been areas of women's skills.

Today, in Britain at least, the traditional role of the midwife is again recognized, and the Royal College of Midwives ensures high standards and training. In most districts, pregnant women are assigned a personal midwife early in their pregnancies whom they consult regularly throughout the nine months. The midwife thus builds up a good personal relationship with the mother-to-be. Whenever possible, this midwife will deliver the baby when it is due: modern midwives are dedicated, and many plan their personal timetables and commitments around the expected delivery dates of their patients to ensure being available when needed. Although most women choose to have babies delivered in the hospital (where the same midwives also work), home births continue to be commonplace and are always an option if the mother prefers, if her health is good, and if there is no reason to expect complications.

Many English midwives, quite legally, use herbal remedies during the various stages of labor, and many labor wards take a very liberal view of what a woman may use during labor to give her comfort; herbal teas may even be accepted in hospitals. After the birth, it is very common for new mothers to be sent home with a tube of marigold cream to ease sore nipples during breastfeeding, while the old folk remedy of cabbage leaves to soothe mastitis has been quoted to me by at least two experienced orthodox midwives as a regular and effective favorite.

Obviously, countries vary, and the cooperation that has developed—and is increasing—in Britain between orthodox practitioners and herbalists is not found everywhere. British herbalists have a formalized and reputable four-year training program in basic medical skills and diagnosis as well as in the therapeutic use of plants. This training reflects a scientific approach to our discipline rather than traditional and intuitive use, although for most practitioners this "art of the herbalist" is soon regarded as an equally vital skill to acquire once they begin to practice. In the United Kingdom, the last few years have seen a greater willingness to embrace holistic principles among orthodox practitioners as well. Doctors no longer want simply to treat physical symptoms, but to see these in the total context of a whole person with emotional and spiritual problems as well. This movement is sometimes referred to as "the greening of medicine."

In the United States, medical herbalism remains "virtually outlawed," to quote American herbalist Michael Tierra. So, one can guess that the use of herbal remedies in midwifery is frowned upon, and there are often legal restrictions on who may assist at a birth as well.

The European herbs recommended by most Western-trained herbalists are familiar garden and wayside plants for use on this side of the Atlantic, and most women have no qualms about dosing themselves with such friendly and everyday brews. Perhaps in the United States it is different. Inevitably, this book reflects a British approach to using herbs in pregnancy and childbirth.

It is important for women to be as honest and open as they can with their physicians about their use of alternative remedies. Some doctors will be more sympathetic to complementary remedies than will others. Try to discuss alternative herbal remedies with your practitioner, gain her viewpoint, and then decide for yourself what is best for you. Modern medicine is often about "magic bullets" and "wonder cures," and we expect our doctors to have a simple solution for all our ills. Using self-help remedies is also about taking responsibility for your own health—and that of your baby—rather than simply accepting whatever orthodox medicine has to offer.

This self-responsibility needs to be vigorously asserted when it comes to some of the routine drug administration used both in childbirth and on newborn babies. In Britain (and probably in the United States as well), there are well-documented cases of drugs given to expel the placenta causing brain damage in an as yet unborn and unexpected twin baby, and of oxytocin injections to speed labor leading to oxygen starvation and brain-damaged infants. Vitamin injections, routine use of antibiotics, and even potentially damaging eyedrops are all regular practices adopted for newborn babies in various parts of the world. Persuading hospital doctors that you and your baby really don't want these treatments can be a challenge.

One decision about your baby's care that you'll want to make well ahead of time is whether to have your baby boy circumcised. Male circumcision—the surgical removal of the foreskin—is regarded as a standard procedure for neonates in the United States as a hygiene measure, to prevent possible painful foreskin infections, and also as a measure to avoid a nonretractable foreskin (phimosis) in later life. Although around 80 to 90 percent of all American males are still circumcised, the figure is very much lower in Europe—only 2 percent of Danish men are circumcised, and around 21,000 boys (about 6 percent) are circumcised each year in the United Kingdom, mainly for religious reasons. The operation is extremely painful and can leave babies deeply traumatized—some people suggest it may cause them relationship problems as they grow older.

At birth, the foreskin is still developing and is naturally intractable; around 40 percent of boy babies still have an intractable foreskin at one year, and 10 percent still have the condition at three years of age. In most cases, this phimosis resolves quite naturally, and a Danish study suggests that by mid-teens barely 1 percent of boys have any foreskin problems. In Europe, a number of alternatives to circumcision are now offered for this condition, including prepuceplasty, a conservative alternative aimed at preserving the foreskin.

There really is no reason to have babies routinely circumcised. Cases of foreskin infection are rare in Europe, and the operation is also regarded as not without risk—excessive bleeding is a common complication, as is sepsis, too much removal of the skin, and possible permanent damage to the penis. There are even documented clinical reports of children whose penises have been so badly mutilated that amputation and "gender rearrangement" with female hormones have been prescribed.

Researchers also suggest that removing the foreskin can interfere with later sex life, because the foreskin is not simply a flap of skin but a double layer of sensitive tissue. The mucous membrane is packed with highly specialized nerves and blood vessels that are believed to enhance the sensory experience during sexual intercourse.

One U.K. critic has described standard North American circumcision as a "big bread and butter money spinner" for the medical profession as well as a "primary source of human skin to be grown on in the lab for grafting." Others suggest that circumcision of a healthy child actually breaches ten articles of the U.N. Convention of the Rights of the Child. There is also a growing lobby against the operation among the Jewish community (who mostly, along with Muslims, still regard circumcision as a necessary religious ritual).

Educating yourself about the various procedures that most hospitals and doctors in the United States regard as standard for new mothers and newborns is the best way to ensure that you and your baby get exactly the care that you want and need.

About This Book

This book is divided into eleven chapters. The first, "Planning for Childbirth," looks at preparation for pregnancy, covering health problems before pregnancy, conception, and infertility. The second, "Pregnancy," provides a monthly progress report on developments during the pregnancy, and includes information about diet, exercise, and massage. The next two chapters address the ailments associated with pregnancy itself, examining herbal remedies for both minor ills and discomforts, such as heartburn and constipation, as well as more serious conditions such as preeclampsia. Those health problems calling for professional help are clearly indicated; in some cases, these may be life threatening for mother or fetus, so do not delay seeking professional help. Most problems in pregnancy are minor, however, and will respond well to simple herbal remedies. In all cases, if symptoms persist for more than a couple of days or if the condition appears to worsen, seek medical help immediately.

The next chapters cover childbirth itself and the immediate postnatal period, and include herbs to help ease labor pains and deal with problems such as depression and perineal tears.

Chapter 7 is devoted to breast-feeding issues and is followed by a chapter on herbs for common health problems in new babies. Chapter 10 is a comprehensive *materia medica* listing all the plants mentioned in the book, and chapter 11 gives general guidelines on how to use the herbs in simple homemade remedies.

Herbal remedies can be effective and healing, but they are often also very potent. They should always be respected for the powerful drugs they are, and this is never more important than during pregnancy. Many herbs contain chemicals that can cross the placental barrier, and others act as uterine stimulants and can cause premature contractions. As with all medication, try to avoid taking high or regular doses of herbs during the first three months of pregnancy, use minimal doses for as short a time as possible, and avoid any unnecessary remedies. A full list of plants to avoid during pregnancy is included in chapter 9. It is also best to avoid most of these plants during the preconception phase. Pregnancy testing kits may be more efficient these days, but there are still likely to be a few weeks between fertilization of the ovum and full realization by the woman that she is pregnant, and potentially toxic remedies need to be avoided during this crucial time. If you are trying to become pregnant, avoid these high-risk herbs at all times.

Note: In general, "oil" refers to the essential oil. Use of an infused oil is always specified as such. Herbal quantities in teas are for dried herbs. Unless otherwise specified, doses should be repeated up to three times a day. Follow the standard doses given in chapter 11, "How to Prepare Herbal Remedies," unless other quantities are specified.

Herbs for a Healthy Pregnancy

1
Planning for Childbirth

In her classic book, *Wise Woman Herbal for the Childbearing Year*, Susun Weed describes this crucial period as being thirteen months long—the two months before conception, the nine months of pregnancy, and the two months following the birth. Throughout this period the mother's health and well-being have a direct effect on her growing baby. One can easily extend this thirteen-month year to at least eighteen months, adding an extra preconceptual month and, as many women would agree, at least a full six months after the baby is born to return completely to normal. After the birth, a woman's body can take at least three months, sometimes longer, to return to its prepregnancy state. It will take many more years for the child to lose his or her total dependence on the mother.

Before conception it is essential to be as fit—both physically and emotionally—as possible; health during pregnancy is now recognized as having a significant long-term effect on the future of the new child, and many chronic ills of our age are now associated with poor fetal care.

In traditional Chinese medicine, the energy that we receive at birth from our parents is called congenital *qi* (vital energy) and inherited *jing* (essence). This built-in store of energy has to last throughout our lives—it cannot be added to or expanded, only supplemented by other sorts of energy derived from living a healthy lifestyle and producing the right kind of postnatal *jing* from suitable nutrients or by developing *qi* with the help of suitable herbs and *qi*-building exercises (as in traditional *qigong* therapy). That special original *jing* cannot be altered and will slowly diminish during our life spans.

These two aspects are traditionally referred to as the "former heaven" and the "latter heaven"; the "former heaven" reflects inherited energy and the "latter" that which we can acquire through good nutrition and beneficial exercise.

A healthy preconceptual period will, in this philosophy, ensure a healthy baby with strong *jing* to guarantee a healthy and long life.

Preconception and Conception

Any woman trying to conceive needs to ensure that she eats a healthy diet with sufficient minerals, vitamins, and other nutrients and, whenever possible, needs to avoid artificial food additives, pollutants, and genetically modified foods by choosing organically grown produce. It is also essential to quit smoking and reduce alcohol intake at least three months before trying to conceive.

The same advice applies to men: researchers have shown in a number of trials that food additives and common industrial chemicals can lower sperm counts and reduce male fertility. Over the past twenty years, male sperm counts have typically fallen by 2 percent a year. Even household soaps and washing powders have been blamed—one study demonstrated that surfactants, used to improve the efficiency of these products, can mimic female hormones and actually become more estrogenlike as they are degraded by bacteria (Lincoln 1994). As these chemicals move through the usual municipal recycled water system—from sewage to purification plant to fresh water supply—they end up in our drinking water and affect male hormone balance. Add to that the waste products from women taking hormone replacement therapy (HRT) or contraceptive pills, and it is clear that men are being exposed to far higher levels of female sex hormones than their fathers or grandfathers ever were. The same chemicals have been implicated as causing infertility among wildlife and even sex changes in fish swimming in estrogen-polluted rivers. The problem is worldwide. Even back in the 1980s, scientists were trying to discover why male alligators hatching from eggs laid around Lake Apopka in Florida had tiny penises and female hormone patterns while the lake's turtles were turning into hermaphrodites.

Apart from drinking water, pollutants and pesticides in our food can also be to blame, so if organically grown produce is not available, peel or wash all fruit and vegetables thoroughly.

Sperm also needs to be kept cool, so tight underpants and trousers that don't allow air to circulate can contribute to infertility problems. If sperm get too hot, they become less active and lack the energy to swim up the vagina to fertilize the waiting egg. Even the ancient Romans appreciated this: a hot bath taken by the man before making love was a simple, popular, and often very effective contraceptive measure.

It takes around twelve weeks for a sperm to grow from its first single cell to full maturity; throughout this period, it is vulnerable to potential damage from external sources. While it is generally accepted that women should not smoke during pregnancy, sperm can also be damaged by cigarettes during this crucial three-month period. One German study has shown a definite link between congenital birth defects and fathers who smoke, so giving up cigarettes at least three months before seriously trying for a baby is a sensible precaution (Schouenborg et al. 1992). Similar research applies to alcohol and also to metal pollutants. To be safe, avoid cooking in aluminum saucepans, eating out-of-date canned foods, or stripping old white paintwork (which might contain lead) during this time.

Both partners should eat as wide and varied a diet as possible, with high levels of beta-carotene and folic acid; deficiencies in both these substances in the three months prior to conception

Tips for the Three Months Before Conception for Mothers- and Fathers-to-Be

- Take an antioxidant supplement including vitamins A, C, and E. Over-the-counter herbal antioxidants are also worth considering, although they are more suitable for men, as they often contain sage or rosemary (which can act as uterine stimulants in high quantities).
- Reduce alcohol consumption to no more than two to three glasses of wine (or the equivalent) each week. Stop smoking.
- Men should take up to 500 mg of vitamin C daily; this will encourage healthy sperm. Eat a couple of oranges each day as well.
- Take zinc supplements or eat plenty of pumpkin seeds, which are rich in this nutrient.
- Drink bottled water instead of tap water to avoid recirculated estrogens. If low sperm count is a major problem, use bottled water for cooking as well.
- Avoid contact with all artificial chemicals, such as cleaning solvents and garden pesticides. Wear protective gloves if you have to handle these substances, and avoid inhaling the fumes.
- Avoid all food additives, especially the hidden ones found in cattle and poultry treated with growth hormones or antibiotics. Eat organically grown foods whenever possible.

have been associated with birth defects. Good sources of these nutrients include apricots, bananas, carrots, citrus fruit, dates, oats, olives, pineapple, oily fish, shellfish, eggs, liver, and dark leafy green vegetables such as spinach.

Women should also avoid unnecessary medication: this is especially important in the first weeks of pregnancy, a time at which the mother-to-be may not yet realize she has conceived. Unnecessary medication also includes herbs; although most are perfectly safe during pregnancy, many do contain chemicals that can cross the placental barrier and damage the fetus. Some will also stimulate the womb, leading to muscle spasms and possible miscarriage (see "Herbs to Avoid in Pregnancy" on page 81).

Certain foods also need to be approached with caution if there is any chance that you may be pregnant; for example, soft, unpasteurized cheeses can be high in bacteria such as *Salmonella* and *Listeria*—no problem for the healthy but now known to be potential hazards for the young fetus. Meat contaminated with particular strains of the bacteria *E. coli*—typically inadequately cooked burgers or infected processed meats—can lead to kidney damage that will also threaten the fetus.

Excess tea, coffee, and other caffeine-containing drinks such as maté or cola also need to be limited as they can inhibit the absorption of certain nutrients, including zinc, which is important for the immune system and helps protect sperm against free-radical damage. Caffeine-rich drinks can also lead to palpitations and heart irregularities. Drink no more than 2 cups of caffeine-containing drinks each day.

Dealing with Infertility

For many women the struggle to conceive becomes an all-consuming preoccupation. Modern fertilization techniques can be very successful but are often expensive, invasive, and unpleasant, and require dedication from both partners.

Herbs can help improve general health and readiness for conception and can be generally supportive, but they are not a magic formula with guaranteed success. Nor can herbs help the many mechanical causes of infertility, such as a retroverted uterus or blocked fallopian tubes. Professional herbal treatment can help if endometriosis, chronic cystitis, ovarian cysts, or candidiasis are interfering with conception.

I remember one patient named Sally, then in her late thirties, who sought herbal treatment for chronic nasal catarrh and phlegm. She and her husband had tried to conceive for ten years before adopting a baby girl, two years earlier. The catarrh was related to an underlying problem with candidiasis, and after three months of herbal treatment and a low-yeast diet Sally had improved so much that we phased out the herbal medication. Two months later I received a telephone call—to her very great surprise, she was pregnant. Her husband was overjoyed, and their little daughter was equally delighted when a baby brother arrived in due course.

Where there is no apparent reason for infertility, a healthy diet and lifestyle, as well as relaxed lovemaking, can help. Stress, tension, and tiredness—especially common for working women who may already have reached their midthirties—will certainly hinder conception. Concern that the biological clock is ticking and time is running out simply adds to the emotional pressure. Equally, there is often a "right time" to conceive—when both partners are ready, emotionally and physically, for the joys and trials of parenthood. We all know of cases where couples try for years for a child before accepting the fact that they are unlikely to have a family of their own and so set off on some new work project or major lifestyle change to reflect their planned childless future, only to find that within months the woman has conceived and they are once more reassessing their plans.

Maintaining a relaxed attitude and not worrying about conception are often far more effective than an endless round of invasive treatments.

In Europe, approximately 12 to 14 percent of couples are infertile; in 40 percent of cases the problem is male, rather than female, infertility. As well as following the advice given on pages 2–3 for avoiding too many estrogenlike substances, try tonic herbs to improve male fertility: ginseng, saw palmetto, damiana, and winter cherry can all help, but only in conjunction with a healthy diet and unpolluted drinking water. Most of these tonics are readily available in over-the-counter tablets and capsules, so take the recommended dosage (usually one or two tablets equivalent to 600 to 1,000 milligrams daily) of any of them. Alternatively, use damiana in herbal tea (2 teaspoons per cup) twice a day.

As a general tonic for the female reproductive system, drink 2 cups of an herbal infusion containing equal amounts of red clover flowers, stinging nettles, lady's mantle, and marigold petals (2 teaspoons of the mix per cup) daily. Add a pinch of peppermint to improve the flavor if necessary. Alternatively, take 5 drops of false unicorn root tincture daily in warm water. *Dong quai* capsules (600 milligrams daily) will also help to stimulate the reproductive system. Do not take *dong quai* if there is a chance you may be pregnant; limit treatment only to the ten days following the start of menstrual bleeding. Chaste tree berries (10 drops of tincture in water taken each morning) can help to normalize the menstrual cycle and so assist you to match sexual intercourse with your fertility peak (generally fourteen to seventeen days after the start of a period).

If a low-grade yeast infection and mild bladder infections seem to be affecting fertility, try to avoid orthodox antibiotics or antifungals. Use a clove of garlic in cooking daily (or take a garlic supplement) as well as 400 milligrams of echinacea in capsules or 1 teaspoon of echinacea tincture in water each day. Seek professional help in more severe cases.

2
Pregnancy

Monthly Progress: The Fetus

After three months of healthy preconception comes the forty weeks of pregnancy and all that it entails. The time is usually divided into three distinct phases or trimesters: early, middle, and late.

Early Pregnancy: Weeks One to Twelve

During this time, the initial embryo grows rapidly into the established fetus. By week twelve, all the major organs are formed. This is the period of highest risk of damage and abnormalities, and early diagnosis of the pregnancy is essential so that the mother can be certain to avoid any destructive toxins.

Malformed fetuses will often abort naturally during this time: up to one in five pregnancies in developed countries end in miscarriage, and the figure is much higher in the Third World.

During this period, the embryo changes dramatically into a recognizable fetus as the fertilized egg divides and grows. Implantation of the fertilized egg in the womb lining generally takes place by the sixth day, and by the sixteenth day the tiny embryo is discernible from its nutrient egg sac, with the cells around the head area proliferating most rapidly. Limb buds appear during the fourth and fifth weeks of the pregnancy, and by the end of the fifth week these are clearly identifiable as three separate components that will eventually form the arms, forearms, and hands or the thighs, legs, and feet.

After the second month, the embryo is generally referred to as a fetus. By then the placenta has formed and the fetus has a clearly recognizable face with early eyes, external ears, and a cleft that will become the mouth.

Middle Pregnancy: Weeks Twelve to Fourteen

Over the next twelve weeks, the fetus continues to grow and the body organs mature. The early yolk sac shrinks as the placenta takes over the supply of nutrients; eventually this will expand to cover approximately one-sixth of the womb's area. By five months, the fetus looks just like a tiny baby; the internal organs gradually mature and external features take on their characteristic shapes.

Typically the pregnancy is "visible" as a growing abdominal bump from about four months.

Late Pregnancy: Weeks Twenty-Four to Thirty-Eight

During the late stage of pregnancy, birth is imminent. The baby grows more slowly through this period, and the greatest effort goes into perfecting the internal organs and their physiology. Today premature babies are generally considered to have a reasonable chance of survival from about twenty-eight weeks, although at this stage many internal organs are still immature and the baby will probably need help with breathing and require intravenous feeding.

The placenta reaches its maximum efficiency between thirty-two and thirty-six weeks and, about six weeks before the baby is due to be born, starts to degenerate so that by the time the baby arrives, its supply of nutrients has become seriously depleted and independent life is essential.

During the final weeks, the fetus—which has been happily moving around in its sea of amniotic fluid—gradually settles into position within the womb, head down and ready for the birth.

Monthly Progress: The Mother

For the mother, these stages are marked by her own changing body shape and increased activity from the growing fetus—the traditional "quickening of the womb" usually felt from around four months as the baby becomes more active. In some pregnancies this characteristic fluttering may occur two months earlier; other women go through a completely normal pregnancy and produce a healthy child without ever really being aware of the baby's movements.

For most women, the first sign of pregnancy is a missed period. A few, however, do continue with light and irregular menstruation for the first four or five months of the pregnancy (usually with markedly reduced flow), so this is not always a guaranteed indicator. Standard urine testing generally confirms a pregnancy at four weeks, although over-the-counter testing kits often indicate a positive result well before that.

Early diagnosis is essential. In the days before efficient pregnancy testing kits, women were far more familiar with the changes in their own bodies that could suggest a pregnancy. Early physical signs of pregnancy include increased breast tenderness, with some enlargement and change in color of the nipple and areola (the area around the nipple) after two months. The areola also becomes more nodular. There is often increased urination and usually an obvious thickening of the waist.

In the early stages of pregnancy women often feel extremely tired, with difficulty concentrating and increased emotional sensitivity; tears come easily and it can be difficult to organize everyday mental activities. Pregnant women may also be restless, wanting to change position frequently from sitting to lying. Morning sickness or vague feelings of nausea may start from the fourth week, and there is often a decrease in appetite.

For many women, the first trimester is the most difficult. The pregnancy is not obvious, so there is little sympathy from others and not much likelihood of being offered a seat on crowded trains or buses, no matter how tired or disoriented one feels. Other women find this time passes very easily with few physical signs or discomforts associated with the pregnancy. In older women or those with an erratic menstrual cycle it is common to be totally unaware of the growing baby until well into the fifth month. On rare occasions, the baby's arrival may even be completely unexpected after the mother has spent several months dieting to avoid what she thought was "middle-aged spread."

By the start of the second trimester, usually around the fourteenth week, these initial discomforts begin to ease. Women at this stage often feel very energetic and look remarkably well—the traditional "bloom" of pregnancy. The growing baby becomes more obvious, and, with the worst risks of miscarriage or abnormalities past, this is often the time women most enjoy. They can start planning the birth, equipping the nursery, and generally letting the world know that a new baby is on the way.

Health problems at this stage are more closely linked to the demands of the increasing bulk in the distended abdomen and the hormonal changes associated with pregnancy. Metabolic, respiratory, and heart rates all change to meet the baby's demands. There is a greater volume of body fluids so the heart must work harder to pump the additional blood around the body. The kidneys also have to go into overtime to filter and cleanse this extra fluid. The extra volume can contribute to varicose veins. Changes in hormones help the ligaments to soften and relax so that joints become more flexible and expandable in readiness for the birth; this can contribute to backache. The hormonal softening also slows the digestive tract; food takes longer to pass through so absorption of essential nutrients is improved, but the chance of constipation greatly increases as well. As the baby grows and becomes more active, there can often be a great deal of laborious heaving, which often interferes with a restful night's sleep.

Apart from all these physical changes, there are plenty of emotional upheavals as well. There is often the shock of realizing—especially with a first baby—that very soon all those freedoms that modern women take for granted will suddenly be curtailed by the arrival of this totally dependent new being. Many women underestimate just how much work is involved in caring for a new baby. Trying to gain some insights into the demands ahead by talking to other mothers can often help avert some of the emotional problems that can follow the birth.

There are family adjustments to be made as well. Older children can often be extremely jealous of a new arrival and need to be encouraged to take an interest and join in the anticipation and enthusiasm for the newcomer. Partners, too, can feel neglected—especially if it is a first baby and a close relationship seems to be threatened by the imminent arrival of a third member.

Lovemaking During Pregnancy

Although lovemaking during pregnancy has historically been regarded as taboo in many cultures, today most practitioners take a more liberal approach because, from a medical point of view, sexual intercourse in pregnancy is perfectly safe. The fetus is well protected by its amniotic fluid, and the womb is well away from the vagina. Intercourse may lead to occasional spotting, as the blood vessels around the cervix have a greater blood supply during pregnancy than at other times. If this occurs, it is best to inform your doctor and avoid deep penetration for a while. Women prone to miscarriage are generally advised to avoid full sexual contact for the first trimester until the pregnancy is well established.

Many women find that pregnancy increases their sexual feelings—especially since there is no need to worry about contraception—and they may experience full orgasm, perhaps for the first time. Others want to avoid sexual relations, especially during the first few weeks, when they may be feeling especially tired and emotionally unsettled.

As long as lovemaking remains gentle and relaxed, it can prove beneficial for both parents and baby, creating a warm, loving energy for the entire family and a comfortable feeling of oneness. The old wives' tradition that lovemaking will also bring on an overdue birth is also not entirely lacking in validity; intercourse can often stimulate labor (but only when the baby is due) since the prostaglandins in semen can help to soften the cervix, providing a quite natural preparation for the birth.

These days it is common for men to attend prebirth classes with their partners, and they are encouraged to become active participants, helping with breathing exercises and learning simple massage techniques. Older children can help too—massaging mommy's tummy or listening to the baby's heartbeat is a good way to encourage a growing relationship.

Diet

Healthy eating in pregnancy is essential, not just to minimize potential pollutants as with the preconception diet but to provide a balanced and sufficient mix of nutrients for the growing baby.

The old tradition of "eating for two" is something of an exaggeration and can contribute to excessive and unnecessary weight gain during pregnancy. Rather, the mother should eat for "one and a little bit." Weight gain in pregnancy is closely monitored by doctors, and any excess will soon be identified.

Although some perfectly normal women gain very little weight during pregnancy (10 to 12 pounds total), more typically by the end of the pregnancy the combined weight of baby, additional body fat, and fluids could be as much as 34 to 35 pounds, although the average is likely to be around 22 to 24 pounds (see Table 2.1 for the typical makeup of this weight gain).

There is likely to be little significant weight gain during the first ten to twelve weeks of the pregnancy, but after that, weight increases by about one pound a week.

Pregnant women need a minimum of 2,200 calories per day—more if they have a physically active job or lifestyle. Typically,

TABLE 2.1 *Typical Makeup of Average Weight Gain During Pregnancy*

Source of Weight	Pounds
Baby	7–9
Placenta	1.5–2
Amniotic fluid	1.5–2
Increase in the womb	2
Additional breast tissue	2
Additional blood	3–4
Additional stored fat	4–5

daily food intake should increase by no more than 20 percent, although there is additional demand for calcium, zinc, magnesium, folic acid, vitamin C, and the B-complex vitamins. Good sources of these are given in Table 2.2. If necessary, take a multivitamin or mineral supplement to boost intake, after consulting your doctor.

The daily diet should include 2 ounces of pure protein. That amount of protein is found in roughly two chicken legs, four eggs, ½ pound of fish, or 10 ounces of cooked lentils. Strict vegetarians who avoid eggs and dairy products need to be especially careful to ensure an adequate protein intake, as the mix of amino acids needed to create human proteins requires combining grains and legumes each day; for example, eating lentil soup with a piece of whole-grain bread or chickpeas with rice or pasta. Vegans are also at risk for vitamin B_{12} deficiency and may need to take supplements.

Another useful recommendation for everyone—not just pregnant women—is to eat at least five portions of fruit, salad, or vegetables each day. These could include, for example, a piece of

TABLE 2.2 *Dietary Sources of Essential Minerals and Vitamins*

CALCIUM	ZINC	MAGNESIUM	FOLIC ACID	VITAMIN B	VITAMIN C
Sardines	Meat	Nuts	Eggs	Whole grains	Most fruits—especially kiwis and citrus
Beans	Nuts	Shrimp	Whole grains	Meat	
Cereals	Chicken	Soybeans	Spinach	Fish	Green vegetables
Nuts	Egg yolk	Leafy green vegetables	Broccoli	Peas/beans	
Dairy Products	Green peas		Collards	Lentils	Potatoes
Salmon	Shellfish	Whole grains	Root vegetables	Brown rice	Rose hips
Seaweeds*	Whole grains		Oysters	Leafy green vegetables	Bell peppers
Sprouted seeds	Turnips		Salmon	Eggs	
Kale	Potatoes		Dates	Bananas	
Sesame seeds	Carrots		Mushrooms	Avocados	
Broccoli	Pumpkin seeds			Nuts/seeds	

*Seaweeds are rich in sodium so they should be avoided by those with a tendency for high blood pressure.

fruit or fresh fruit juice at breakfast, salad and a piece of fruit at lunch, and two servings of vegetables with the evening meal.

Foods to Avoid

Certain foods should be avoided. Some nutritionists now suggest that the seeds of coronary heart disease are sown not only in early childhood but in the womb, so eating too much saturated fat and sugar during pregnancy could have a damaging long-term effect on your offspring. It is best, therefore, to reduce intake of sausages, burgers, pastries, and candies during pregnancy.

Too much salt in susceptible women can cause fluid retention and increase the risk of elevated blood pressure. The recommended maximum daily salt intake is roughly equivalent to 1 level teaspoon; most people eat far more, thanks to excessive use of salt in convenience foods and "junk" meals. Alcohol and caffeine-containing drinks (for example, tea, coffee, or cola) can interfere with nutrient absorption, while alcohol also has been associated with birth defects.

Excessive vitamin A is another cause of fetal deformities; some nutritionists go so far as to recommend cutting out liver and liver pâtés during pregnancy. Liver is, however, such a good source of other valuable nutrients that total avoidance seems rather excessive—an occasional liver dish will do little harm.

As during the preconception diet, continue to avoid unpasteurized milk or cheeses as well as soft or blue cheeses; these may contain *Listeria* bacteria that may damage the fetus. Prepared salad packs have also been associated with *Listeria* poisoning, so avoid these as well. Raw eggs or runny yolks can be a source of *Salmonella* contamination. Give up rare steaks for the duration; undercooked meat and poultry may be contaminated with *E. coli* and can also lead to toxoplasmosis, yet another potential cause of fetal damage. Wear gloves when cleaning the cat's litter tray or handling soil that may be contaminated with animal droppings; these too can be a source of toxoplasmosis. In healthy adults toxoplasmosis generally causes little more than enlarged lymph nodes for a few days, but during pregnancy it can be transmitted to the fetus and cause blindness and mental abnormalities.

There are also many herbs to avoid (see page 81). Don't take unnecessary pharmaceutical drugs, including over-the-counter analgesics or cough mixtures. Check with your doctor before taking any medication.

Cravings and Anemia

Be prepared for those unexpected food cravings often associated with pregnancy. These have been linked with iron deficiency, so rather than being simply amused by sudden urges for pickles, lumps of coal, or late-night binges on corned beef sandwiches, have your hemoglobin levels checked to identify any early signs of iron-deficiency anemia.

Good dietary sources of iron include beef, sardines, eggs, dried fruits (especially apricots, figs, and prunes), almonds, blackstrap molasses, brewer's yeast, cocoa, whole-grain bread, beetroot, broccoli, leafy green vegetables, seaweeds, and sprouted seeds such as mung beans and alfalfa. Vitamin C is needed for efficient iron absorption, so combine these foods with citrus fruit or the vitamin C–rich foods listed earlier.

Exercise

Giving birth is an energetic, physical process demanding stamina and flexibility. In traditional societies, where women lead far more active lives than in our sedentary Western world, there is little need for increased exercise to get ready for birth; their bodies are already well prepared for the effort.

For many Western women, however, additional exercise is essential. This should not be energetic aerobics or strenuous workouts in the gym. Rather, exercise is needed to help calm and center the mother, allowing her to concentrate energies on the growing baby while maximizing the suppleness of her limbs and ligaments in preparation for the birth.

Increased progesterone levels during pregnancy are responsible for the natural softening of ligaments to create a more flexible skeleton; this additional suppleness makes yoga exercises ideal—those apparent contortions become simple for pregnant women as they find they can move their bodies more easily than before.

Attending yoga classes is generally the best way to get started, especially for novices. Qualified yoga teachers are very familiar with the needs of pregnant women and will often recommend a suitable routine. If there is no convenient class in your area, the exercises illustrated and described in books such as Sandra Jordan's *Yoga for Pregnancy* show easy step-by-step movements.

One of the simplest techniques—common to both yoga and *qigong*—is "simple standing," which will help combat general tiredness and insomnia as well as improve what is generally referred to as "grounding" (a sense of oneness with the natural world around us). Stand upright naturally with feet about 12 inches apart in a well-balanced position and raise the crown of the head gently while keeping the body relaxed and comfortable. Some teachers suggest imagining an invisible thread connecting the top of your head to the sky which very gently pulls you upright without any tension or strain. With your mouth closed, eyelids drooping, and relaxed shoulders, concentrate on a point below your navel. Serious students of *qigong* will stand in this position for many hours concentrating totally on the energy center below the navel and not permitting their minds to wander at all. In pregnancy, however, standing still for longer than a few minutes can easily make one feel lightheaded or dizzy, so continue only for as long as the position is completely comfortable and tension free.

Swimming is also extremely beneficial in pregnancy—the buoyancy of the water is both soothing and supporting and can help one exercise without undue strain. A gentle splash around the pool once or twice a week—more if you find it helpful—is ideal, but don't attempt overenergetic strokes or intense diving routines.

Try to devote an hour a day to your exercise and breathing routines, ideally choosing a time when the rest of the family will not interrupt you and you can be quiet and peaceful. Begin with a warm bath to relax the muscles, and don't eat for an hour before your exercise session. Start by sitting comfortably—either cross-legged on the floor, kneeling, or upright on a chair, whichever is best for you—with your hands placed palm down on your lower abdomen. Breathe in slowly through your nose while counting up to five. Concentrate on how the breath travels through your body and your abdomen moves gently upward. Hold your breath for a further count of five while concentrating, and then breathe out through the mouth while making a "huu" sound, also to the count of five. Again, concentrate on how your abdomen moves gently downward. If you find it easier to visualize something while breathing, imagine your breath as a wave washing over you before retreating once more. Continue this deep breathing for about five or ten minutes before placing your hands on your knees, palms up and sitting quietly, relaxed for a few minutes more.

Follow your breathing routine with simple standing for a few minutes. Then rest by lying on the floor on your left side with one knee bent and supported by cushions. Now, it's time to try a few simple yoga postures. Typically, this may include kneeling on all fours with knees and palms about 12 inches apart and alternately arching and relaxing the spine while breathing in and out. Full details of these exercises can be found in any good yoga book or, even better, under the guidance of a good yoga teacher. Try to attend a few classes to learn the basic techniques early in your pregnancy (or even better, start yoga before you conceive). Always rest and relax for a few minutes, by lying on the floor as before, in between each yoga posture.

As the pregnancy advances, the baby's weight can often lead to back pain and discomfort. Good posture is important to reduce the strain on the spine. It is also vital to lift heavy objects (or toddlers) correctly. Always bend from the knees rather than the waist when picking up heavy items.

In the final weeks of pregnancy, it is often more comfortable to squat on a low stool so that the hips and thighs are slightly raised; put your stool against a wall to support your back and avoid any of the deep squatting movements in yoga after the thirty-fourth week. Kneeling with widely spread knees in front of a large beanbag or pile of cushions and gradually leaning forward so that the cushions take your weight can bring relief to lower-back tension. This exercise also encourages the baby into the correct position for birth.

Massage

Regular massage is soothing and restorative at any time, but especially in pregnancy, helping to balance energy flows and prevent ill health. In many parts of the East, massage is seen as an essential part of the midwife's skills as she eases the birth and immediate postnatal recovery period.

Although localized aches and pains can often be helped with self-massage, for a more relaxing treatment it is generally preferable for someone else to perform the massage. This can be a very sensual experience for both giver and receiver, and it is well worth encouraging your partner to develop a few basic massage skills. It can be a rewarding experience for the family—including the unborn child—for your partner to gently stroke and caress your growing abdomen, helping to create a calm, loving, and relaxing atmosphere for all of you.

There are many books demonstrating special massage skills for the novice, although gentle stroking and intuitive motions can often be just as comforting and healing. If it feels right, it generally is right. Don't attempt to massage damaged tissue (such as a twisted ankle)—this can often be harmful—and don't massage bare skin with dry hands, as the friction can lead to soreness. Always use about a teaspoon of almond or wheat germ oil (or even sunflower or olive oil from the kitchen if that is all you have) to lubricate your hands. These oils can be scented with essential oils, such as one drop of rose, lavender, or neroli, if you prefer.

As a daily routine, kneel forward onto a pile of cushions that will support your body comfortably and ask your partner to massage your back and shoulders using a gently circular motion to help ease tensions, improve relaxation, and soothe any aches and pains. For approximately ten to fifteen minutes, your partner should gradually work down your back to the buttocks, and end the massage cycle with the thighs.

For abdominal massage, lie comfortably on your side supported by cushions with your partner lying behind you. He can then massage your abdomen with one hand using circular strokes while supporting himself with his other arm.

Self-massage can also be helpful as part of a regular routine. Breast and abdominal massage throughout the pregnancy can help to prevent stretch marks. Massaging the perineal area in the last few weeks will help to prepare for the birth by softening the tissues and improving their stretchability. This is best done after a warm bath with a little almond or wheat germ oil; half kneel with one leg upright to expose the perineum and then gently rub the area with a little oil using the thumb and fingers of one hand.

Massage is also very soothing for small babies. In China, baby massage has long been used by mothers to soothe minor digestive upsets and relax the baby. Usually just the baby's fingers or arms are massaged rather than the sort of full-body massage common with adults. For indigestion, vomiting, and poor appetite, for example, the Chinese mother will simple stroke her finger in a rolling circular motion on the baby's palm—not once or twice but about 200 times. For diarrhea she will rub the palm side of her baby's thumb from tip to base up to 500 times. This massages a specific acupuncture point which helps normalize digestion.

Like regular exercise, massage should become a part of your daily personal pampering routine.

3
Easing the Discomforts of Pregnancy

For many women, pregnancy is a time of great vitality and radiant health; the vast majority of ailments they are likely to suffer are minor, self-limiting discomforts rather than serious threats to long-term health.

Most problems relate to the body's changing hormone levels. The increase in progesterone production is associated with softening ligaments, relaxing muscles, and lubricating membranes—ideal for preparing for childbirth, but causing a variety of possible unpleasant side effects.

Abdominal Pain

The most obvious causes for unexpected pain during pregnancy are

- ectopic pregnancy in the very early stages, which is a clinical emergency (see chapter 4);
- stretching pains, which occur as the ligaments supporting the womb soften;
- abdominal cramps, more common in early pregnancy (see below);
- premature contractions in the late stages of pregnancy; and
- the onset of labor (see chapter 5) or more severe conditions such as placental separation, ruptured uterus, ruptured stomach rectus muscle, kidney inflammation, or appendicitis, all of which must be treated as clinical emergencies.

To ease stretching pains, make a decoction of cramp bark (1 teaspoon per cup) mixed with an equal amount of lemon balm or chamomile infusion (1 teaspoon per cup) and sip in half-cup doses every two or three hours. Alternatively, try a warm bath to which 2 cups of this tea has been added.

Braxton Hicks contractions, associated with transitory tightening of the uterine muscles, are commonplace during weeks twenty to twenty-four. Massaging the abdomen with 2 to 3 drops of lavender oil in a teaspoon of almond oil can bring relief. Also, the warm bath recommended above for the early stretching pains may be helpful.

During the last month, false labor pains (a sort of prelabor contraction) are common. Again, try massaging the abdomen with diluted lavender oil or drink a cup of black haw decoction (1 to 2 teaspoons per cup) mixed with ½ cup of motherwort infusion (1 teaspoon per cup) up to three times daily.

Allergies

Although allergies are certainly not confined to pregnancy, it is a period when they can manifest for the first time. Sensitivity to common allergens, such as dust mites, wheat, dairy products, or detergents, is often increased during pregnancy. This may cause skin rashes or miscellaneous gastric disturbances.

Hay fever can often start with pregnancy, when increased mucous secretions contribute to irritation. Regular hay fever sufferers often find their symptoms become significantly worse at this time; many women who wear contact lenses must revert to eyeglasses during pregnancy, as their eyes become very dry and sore.

Identifying and avoiding irritants is important, although pregnancy is not a time to experiment with extreme exclusion diets. Try to note when symptoms are worse and if there is an obvious food trigger or if symptoms coincide with particular routines, such as washing or housecleaning.

Skin rashes can be eased with marigold and chamomile creams or by using borage juice (from freshly crushed leaves) as a wash. Inhaling the steam from chamomile infusion can also help to ease the worst hay fever symptoms. Simply put a tablespoon of the dried flowers into a basin, pour on boiling water, lean over the basin, and cover both it and your head with a towel. Inhale the steam gently until the mixture cools and then remain in a warm room for twenty to thirty minutes. Stay inside if the weather is cold.

If there is a family history of allergy, try to breast-feed your baby for at least six months. Breast milk will help strengthen the developing immune system and reduce the long-term risk of allergy. Cow's and formula milk mixtures for babies contain proteins that are very different from those in human milk; they can be difficult for immature digestive systems to handle. These will also increase the risk of allergies in later life. If there is a history of dairy sensitivity in your family (generally associated with eczema and asthma), you should also avoid drinking cow's milk or eating other milk products while breast-feeding. Use diluted goat's milk or soy milk as a substitute, but don't overdo, as these too may trigger allergic reactions. See the list of calcium-containing foods in chapter 2 if you are concerned that your diet may be calcium deficient as a result of avoiding dairy products.

Iron-Deficiency Anemia

In order to ensure an adequate blood supply to the placenta to nurture the growing fetus, the volume of blood circulating in the body increases during pregnancy. This volume grows more rapidly than the red blood cells can multiply, so their overall concentration is diluted. The result is a relative reduction in the amount of hemoglobin in a given volume of blood. Hemoglobin is used to carry oxygen to the tissues, so any shortage leaves the body starved for oxygen with fatigue, breathlessness, pallor, insomnia, dizziness, assorted aches and pains, confusion, and reduced resistance to infection—all symptoms of anemia. The problem is most likely to occur in the final weeks of pregnancy when the baby takes a growing proportion of the mother's iron supply.

In pregnancy, a convenient orthodox solution is simply to prescribe supplements containing iron salts (usually ferrous sulphate), but these can lead to constipation and indigestion, bringing a new set of problems. A better solution is to ensure a good supply of iron-rich foods in the diet both in the months before conception and throughout the pregnancy. Building up a good reserve of iron before becoming pregnant is especially important for women prone to heavy periods (one of the most common causes of iron-deficiency anemia).

In addition to a good supply of iron, the body needs various vitamins to ensure efficient absorption: vitamin B_{12}, vitamin C, and folic acid are all important. Strict vegetarians (vegans) can be especially short of vitamin B_{12}, which is found most abundantly in meat, fish, dairy products, eggs, and brewer's yeast; regular supplements might be necessary for this group. Good sources of folic acid include green vegetables, liver, eggs, and whole grains (see chapter 2). High alcohol intake can increase the body's requirements for both folic acid and vitamin C; heavy smokers also tend to suffer from vitamin C deficiency.

It is important to eat plenty of iron-rich foods throughout pregnancy. The list of good sources includes eggs, watercress, dried apricots, spinach, cabbage, beets, chicory, sunflower seeds, alfalfa, currants, cherries, lentils, blackberries, and black currants. For generations, liver was valued as an essential, iron-rich food in pregnancy, although more recently many dietitians warn against its consumption, as liver can contain high levels of vitamin A. Moderate liver intake (ideally from organically reared animals, to reduce chemical pollution) should pose little risk.

Those herbs that are said to "rob the soil," such as stinging nettles, concentrate many important minerals and vitamins in their leaves, including iron. Drink 2 or 3 cups of nettle tea each day using 2 teaspoons of dried herb to a cup of boiling water. Also useful are burdock leaves, skullcap, dandelion leaves, kelp, rosehips, and hawthorn leaves. Because these have a number of other physiological effects, they should be used in moderation as a source of iron—no more than 4 cups of each per week. Watercress, dandelion leaves, rosehips, and black currants all contain both vitamin C and iron for optimal absorption.

Caffeine-containing drinks (for example, coffee, tea, and cola) inhibit iron absorption.

Backache

Backache is extremely common in pregnancy. It is caused not only by the growing fetus and the unaccustomed shift in the mother's center of gravity but also because increased progesterone levels soften the tendons and ligaments, relaxing the spine's usual support.

Good posture, a firm (not necessarily hard) mattress, and a comfortable upright chair to support the back are all commonsense precautions. Simple yoga exercises—such as getting down on your hands and knees and alternately arching your back, like a cat, and then relaxing as you breathe in and out—can often help. Regular rest in the last three months is also important. Follow the general guidelines on posture and lifting given in the section on exercise in chapter 2. Lack of magnesium and calcium can also contribute to the problem, so be sure you are getting enough in your diet (see chapter 2).

A good soak in a bath containing 5 drops of lavender oil or a cup of strained chamomile tea will ease back pain. Persuade your partner to massage a little of the same oils (2 to 3 drops of either of these oils in a teaspoon of almond oil) gently into the lower back area, night and morning; add 1 drop of ginger or black pepper oil to the mix if the pain is particularly acute. If you have some infused St. John's wort oil, use that as a base for your massage mix instead of almond or wheat germ oil; it will help relieve pain and irritation in the nerve endings. A hot compress soaked in St. John's wort tea will also bring relief. Internally, St. John's wort and chamomile tea can also help. Use 1 teaspoon of each to a cup of infusion, up to three times a day.

Bladder and Kidney Problems

Increased blood flow to the uterus and growing fetus in early pregnancy causes an increased frequency in urination, often one of the earliest indications of pregnancy. The frequency generally eases after the fourth month of pregnancy but returns in the latter stages as the baby's head starts to press against the bladder.

Urinary tract infections and cystitis are common in pregnancy and affect around one-fifth of expectant mothers; the cause is generally related to stagnant urine collecting in the bladder as raised progesterone levels lead to a relaxation in muscle tone.

An infusion of equal parts of uva-ursi, couch grass, and cornsilk (1 teaspoon of the mix per cup, three times a day) can help in mild cases. A useful alternative is to take these herbs powdered in capsules (widely available in health food stores and some pharmacies). Take 1 teaspoon of echinacea tincture in water as well if the infection becomes more acute. Drink plenty of liquid to flush out the system: use water or diluted (50/50) apple juice and drink at least a quart daily. Cranberry juice also helps combat urinary and bladder infections. Drink a glass of the unsweetened juice four to five times daily.

Good hygiene is important. Wash yourself after urinating using 2 drops of tea tree oil to ½ pint of warm water and gently pat dry.

Breathlessness

Breathlessness with even mild exertion is quite common in pregnancy. If it occurs at rest or during normal physical movements, however, it can suggest iron-deficiency anemia, dietary deficiency, or too great a weight gain, so do mention it to your doctor.

You can improve stamina by regular exercise, especially swimming—try a gentle breaststroke once or twice a week. Regular, calm deep breathing will also help normalize erratic breathing patterns. Follow the routines given earlier in chapter 2, in the section on exercise.

Carpal Tunnel Syndrome

Excessive edema in pregnancy can contribute to carpal tunnel syndrome, common in pregnancy. The swelling caused by fluid retention puts pressure on the nerves and blood vessels that pass through the bony wrist canal (known as the carpal tunnel), and the result can be numbness, tingling, or pain in the hands and lower arm. This can be quite severe at times. When the condition occurs in older women, surgery is often recommended.

Carpal tunnel syndrome in pregnancy will generally resolve reasonably quickly after the birth when fluid levels return to normal. Massage can help—try rubbing your wrist from the base of the thumb to the edge of the wrist and then repeat from the base of the inner hand to the opposite side of the wrist.

Cramp bark decoction can bring relief taken both internally (1 teaspoon per cup up to three times daily) or used to soak a hot compress wrapped around the wrist. Alternatively, use black haw bark (which has a very similar action) or drink a tea containing equal parts of hawthorn, chamomile, and passion flower (1 teaspoon of the mix per cup).

Some studies suggest that carpal tunnel syndrome is associated with vitamin B_6 deficiency. There have been adverse reports in recent years of the side effects of excessive vitamin B_6 supplementation, so check with your doctor for the appropriate dosage. Focus on foods containing vitamin B_6, such as meats, fish, egg yolks, whole-grain cereals, bananas, avocados, nuts, and seeds. Red, greasy, scaly facial skin is often a sign of vitamin B_6 deficiency.

Constipation

Raised progesterone levels also lead to relaxation of the muscles in the digestive tract, so there is always a tendency for constipation in pregnancy. As the baby grows there is additional pressure on the large bowel, impeding normal circulation and bowel movements.

As always with constipation, a diet high in fiber is important to provide enough bulky roughage to keep the bowels working; prunes and figs added to oatmeal or muesli (a type of breakfast cereal combining grains, nuts, and fruit) work well as laxatives, as do plenty of fresh apples and lightly cooked vegetables.

A glass of warm water first thing in the morning is a traditional method for stimulating bowel movements. You can also take psyllium husks before breakfast to help lubricate the bowel. Put 1 teaspoon of the husks into a cup of water or juice. Shake briskly and drink immediately. If you cannot swallow this glutinous mixture easily, buy powdered psyllium in capsules and take with a large glass of water. Ample water is important, because the crushed husks will continue to swell in the stomach.

Regular gentle exercise, such as walking, swimming, or cycling, will also help combat constipation.

Many of the most popular herbal laxatives—such as senna, alder, buckthorn, and cascara sagrada—contain potent chemicals called anthraquinone glycosides, which irritate the bowel and act as purgatives. These are best avoided in pregnancy, as the excessive gut spasm they cause may also irritate the uterus. Instead, choose the milder herbal laxatives—dandelion root, butternut, or licorice. Yellow dock also contains anthraquinone glycosides but in a lower concentration than herbs such as senna, so it can be used in moderation for short periods if constipation is severe (although, like the other strong purgatives, it is also best avoided if possible). To make a tea, use 1 teaspoon of dandelion or licorice root per cup of water and drink first thing each morning; add a pinch of powdered ginger or crushed fennel seeds to the mixture to help expel gas and ease any discomfort in your abdomen.

Edema (Fluid Retention)

Fluid retention is common in the later stages of pregnancy, typically manifesting as puffy ankles and hands. The condition is partly related to changes in blood proteins caused by the demands of the growing fetus. In addition, during the last weeks of pregnancy, there is a natural tendency to retain fluid to avoid dehydration during labor and childbirth. Fluid retention is therefore quite normal, and the expectant mother may retain up to 5 quarts of additional fluid. Gravity inevitably sends this fluid downward—hence the focus on hands and ankles—although there may also be facial puffiness, especially in the morning.

Excessive weight gain and hot weather will make things worse. Severe edema can be a sign of preeclampsia, so worsening of the condition calls for rapid medical attention, especially if swelling is associated with headaches or feeling unwell.

Whatever the cause, fluid retention can be extremely tiring and uncomfortable, making movement and exercise an effort. Resting with the legs raised during the day helps dissipate the fluid and relieve local discomfort. Reducing fluid intake or excessive use of diuretics is not the solution; this simply deprives the growing baby of much-needed fluid. Occasional limited use of herbal diuretics—especially during hot weather or in the afternoon and evening when the swelling generally gets worse—can help: drink a cup of dandelion leaf, horsetail, corn silk, or couch grass tea, or process a large handful of fresh cleavers in a food mixer or juicer and take 1 tablespoon of the purée in water, up to three times a day.

Massage can also be beneficial. Add 2 drops of lavender, rose geranium, patchouli, or lemon oil to a teaspoon of almond oil and massage the affected area, directing the massage pressure back toward the heart and against the direction of gravity. The same oils can be added to bathwater.

Fainting and Low Blood Pressure

Although low blood pressure is generally a sign of good health, a sudden drop in pressure can lead to fainting. This is fairly common, especially in early pregnancy. The cause is linked to muscle softening (due to raised progesterone levels) in the leg veins, so the blood tends to pool there (rather than being pumped efficiently by muscle contractions back toward the heart).

Lying on your back for a long period, standing for too long without moving, a hot bath, or extreme heat can all cause faintness. This is not a major problem, although there is always a risk of injury when fainting. Be sure to inform your doctor and have your blood pressure checked.

Keeping the venous muscles moving by alternately contracting and relaxing the leg and buttock muscles when you must stand for any length of time can help; also, lie on your side rather than your back when resting. Sit or lie down immediately at the slightest sign of faintness and try to raise your legs above your head either by bending forward with your head between your knees (not easy in late pregnancy) or putting your legs on a chair while you lie on the floor. Typical early signs of faintness include pallor, sweating, and yawning.

Keep a bottle of Dr. Bach's Rescue Remedy with you and put a few drops on your tongue if you feel faint. Alternatively, keep a little camphor or rosemary oil in a bottle and sniff it. Sniffing camphor will also aid in the circulation. A cup of weak chamomile tea on regaining consciousness can be beneficial as well.

Severe low blood pressure generally needs professional treatment, and many of the herbalist's favorite remedies are potent herbs best avoided during pregnancy. Potassium-rich foods, such as citrus fruits, bananas, nuts, and oatmeal, should be included in the diet. Taking Korean ginseng tablets (600 milligrams) daily for a short period can also help. Add garlic in cooking or drink a daily cup of damiana tea (1 teaspoon of dried herb per cup). Hawthorn, which is usually used for high blood pressure but actually regulates and normalizes the pressure, can also be helpful in mild low blood pressure problems. Drink a cup (1 teaspoon of dried herb per cup) daily.

Fatigue and Emotional Upsets

With all the hormonal and physical changes in the body, it is no wonder that pregnancy is associated with emotional upsets, tiredness, and general stress. This is especially true for older mothers and those trying to juggle work and family commitments with the demands of the growing fetus.

A good diet is essential to avoid unnecessary exhaustion; eat plenty of fresh produce and limit the intake of sugary foods. Tiredness can also be related to iron-deficiency anemia, so have your hemoglobin levels checked. Siberian or American ginseng can provide an energy boost and increase the body's stamina and ability to cope with stress. Korean ginseng is best avoided; it is a very stimulating *yang* tonic that is too strong for pregnant women.

Useful herbal infusions to calm and soothe emotions include skullcap, lemon balm, chamomile, or lime flowers. Make a tea with 1 teaspoon per cup of water (or use a combination), and repeat up to three times daily; alternatively, use 10 to 20 drops of the tincture in water every few hours. The Bach Flower Remedies and Californian Flower Quintessentials listed in the Stress section may also be helpful. A stimulating bath containing 2 to 3 drops of rosemary oil or a cup of damiana infusion will revitalize flagging energy levels.

Pregnancy is a time of great creativity and spiritual awareness as the new life grows, and it is important to include a little bit of something beautiful every day. This could be a walk in the countryside, good music, or plenty of flowers. During pregnancy women often produce exquisite poetry and paintings, drawing on a depth of emotion they didn't know they had. Many women writers claim to produce their best work when pregnant.

It is important to acknowledge these deep spiritual stirrings and creative outbursts and to make time for them. A daily cup of rose petal infusion is ideal to support these feelings.

Heartburn

Heartburn is common at any time, but in pregnancy a combination of high progesterone levels, relaxing muscles, and the growing fetus putting pressure on the stomach makes it even more likely. The stomach's naturally acidic contents are forced back along the digestive tract to create that familiar burning sensation. In extreme cases, part of the stomach itself can be forced up through the diaphragm, leading to a hiatal hernia.

Eating small portions slowly and often, rather than the conventional two or three large meals a day, will help to reduce the risk of an overfilled stomach; avoid eating late at night and steer clear of foods likely to exacerbate the problem such as coffee and fatty or spicy foods. A couple of bricks under the legs at the head of the bed will provide a gentle slope to help prevent acid regurgitation when sleeping. Always bend from the knees, keeping the back straight; never simply double over.

A cup of catmint, lemon balm, or chamomile tea after meals

will help calm the stomach; meadowsweet is ideal to reduce stomach acids—use 10 drops of tincture three times a day or make the dried herb into a tea. Fennel, anise, and spearmint can be used in the same way, but large doses of these should be avoided during pregnancy. Drink these teas only occasionally.

Slippery elm and marshmallow root powder will also soothe the digestive tract. Make a gruel by mixing 1 teaspoon of the powders (either separately or in combination) into a paste with a little water, then fill the cup with hot milk or water. Both herbs are also available in tablet form (take two before each meal), which is convenient when traveling.

Hemorrhoids

Hemorrhoids are a type of varicose vein associated with constipation and straining. They develop much as varicose veins in the legs do, by relaxation and distention of the blood vessels. In pregnancy a combination of raised progesterone levels, constipation, and increased abdominal pressure limiting blood supply can all contribute to the problem.

Obviously it is important to avoid constipation, and regular use of gentle bulking laxatives, such as psyllium husks, can help. Hemorrhoids tend to itch and will bleed easily; in severe cases professional medical help is essential. They're also usually worse in the later stages of pregnancy when the baby's head moves downward to the pelvis, and blood flow through the veins is further restricted.

Cold compresses can ease the itching and mild bleeding. Use a cloth soaked in a diluted tincture (2 teaspoons to a glass of water) or a well-strained infusion (or decoction) of bistort, oak bark, witch hazel, or plantain leaves and apply to the affected area several times a day. Pilewort ointment is specific for hemorrhoids, or use distilled witch hazel or witch hazel ointment and apply regularly.

Hiatal Hernia

A hiatal hernia is caused when part of the stomach is pushed upward through the gap in the diaphragm where the esophagus runs by the bulk of the growing fetus. The problem often disappears after the birth, although it may become a chronic problem in overweight women or if there is repeated childbearing.

Although most hernias are resolved by surgery, doctors are generally reluctant to operate on hiatal hernias; there is a poor success rate and often discomfort and pain are not severe. Typical symptoms are an increase in acid regurgitation, belching, and a sensation that food is "stuck in the gullet." Symptoms are worse when lying down as acid will then flow naturally under gravity from the stomach to the esophagus. As with heartburn, a simple palliative is to raise the head of the bed so that the sufferer is sleeping at an incline and acid remains in the stomach where it belongs.

A cup of carrot juice before meals is a traditional remedy to ease the symptoms, and it is important to avoid very heavy, rich meals or eating last thing at night. Start the day with 1 cup of chamomile infusion (1 teaspoon of dried herb per cup) and drink ½ cup of meadowsweet infusion (1 to 2 teaspoons per cup) every two to three hours during the day to relieve any discomfort. Chewing three or four slippery elm tablets up to four times daily can also relieve the discomfort. Placing cold compresses soaked in chamomile infusion on the upper abdomen may also bring relief.

Hiatal hernia is often associated with obesity, so keeping weight gain during pregnancy to recommended limits is important. It is also more likely to occur if a multiple birth is expected or the baby has a birth weight well above average.

Insomnia

Restless babies, heartburn, frequent urination, and the general awkwardness of turning over in bed all contribute to insomnia, which is very common in the latter stages of pregnancy.

Sleeplessness only becomes a problem when it leaves one feeling tired and drained; for those able to take frequent catnaps during the day, loss of sleep at night is manageable. Staying calm and relaxed rather than worrying about the inability to sleep is essential. A thermos of a suitable herbal tea taken to bed at night and sipped during periods of wakefulness can help. Otherwise, be prepared to get up, sit in a chair for a few minutes, and listen to some favorite soothing music before heading back to bed.

Useful herbs for insomnia include chamomile, skullcap, passion flower, St. John's wort, and lavender. They can be used in any combination to suit your taste; use 1 teaspoon of the mix to a cup of water to make an infusion, and drink it thirty minutes before bedtime, repeating during the night if necessary. It is best to vary the mixture regularly, as repeated doses can become less effective. Alternatively, you can mix tinctures of these same herbs together and take a maximum of 1 teaspoon of the combination in a little warm water before bedtime.

As in any case of insomnia, it is also best to avoid large meals late at night, limit intake of black tea, coffee, or cola drinks after about 6:00 P.M., and take a relaxing bath—with 2 to 3 drops of lavender or orange blossom (neroli) oil or a cup of strained lemon balm or chamomile tea—half an hour before bed.

Leg Cramps

Leg cramps in pregnancy are related to an imbalance in the body's natural calcium and sodium salt levels and poor circulation caused by the demands of the growing fetus. Usually the leg muscles are affected, although abdominal cramps are also common, especially in the early stages, and they can be extremely uncomfortable.

Rubbing the affected muscle vigorously can ease the cramp. Alternatively, use a warm compress soaked in cramp bark decoction or the tincture diluted in warm water (2 teaspoons to 1 pint of warm water) and hold it against the affected area until the pain eases. If cramping is a problem at night, take a vacuum flask containing the hot decoction and a washcloth to the bedroom so that you can assemble the compress at night with minimum effort.

Eat plenty of calcium-rich foods, such as almonds, blackstrap molasses, broccoli, dried figs, leafy greens, legumes, sardines (with the bones and skin), and watercress. Sesame seeds are also a good source of calcium, so sprinkle them on salads or use tahini (sesame paste) as an alternative to peanut butter. Herbs, too, can help to boost the body's mineral levels to help avoid cramps; horsetail juice (2 teaspoons in water up to three times a day) is useful or make a stinging nettle infusion (1 teaspoon per cup, two to three times daily).

Massaging the legs with 2 to 3 drops of lavender oil in 1 teaspoon of almond oil before bed can also counter any tendency for cramping pains at night. Drinking ½ cup of cramp bark and hawthorn berry decoction (1 teaspoon of each per cup) up to four times a day can also help.

Morning Sickness

For many women, morning sickness is the first indication of pregnancy. The problem generally starts around the fourth week of pregnancy and will usually ease by the fourteenth; it is often accompanied by general lethargy and tiredness. Although morning sickness most commonly occurs for a few minutes on rising, it can actually happen at any time of day and is also prevalent in early evening.

In some rare cases it can be an almost constant problem and extend through much of the nine months. Researchers have found that ginger is extremely effective even in these very severe cases where fluid loss and debility become major problems and hospitalization may be necessary. Up to 1 gram of ginger per dose has been used quite safely in hospital trials, although it is still common to find orthodox practitioners advising against the use of ginger in any form at all during pregnancy, citing the uterine-stimulating activity of related species (though not ginger) as their reasons for caution. The sorts of doses of ginger used for treating minor morning sickness at home fall well short of the hospital trial and can be regarded as quite safe.

There are numerous theories about the cause of morning sickness: some blame low blood sugar; others talk of increased progesterone levels activating the vomiting centers of the brain. In Chinese theory, early pregnancy can be associated with liver imbalance related to changing blood flows, which is believed to lead to nausea. In Chinese terms, nausea is often seen as evidence of irregular energy flows; herbs such as bitter orange are used for sickness in China because they are believed to "reverse the flow of qi (vital energy)," sending it safely back downward.

Many herbs are recommended for morning sickness. One of the most widely cited is black horehound (10 drops of tincture in a little water on rising); however, many women find the smell of this herb even more nauseating than the morning sickness itself, so it is not suitable for everyone.

It's generally best to try a variety of remedies; what works one morning may prove ineffective another day. A simple approach is to dilute 2 teaspoons of a variety of herbal tinctures with an equal amount of water and store each of them in separate dropper bottles. Then take 4 to 5 drops of one of the remedies on the tongue before rising or at the first sign of nausea. Repeat with an effective herb as necessary, and switch to an alternative remedy as soon as one seems to lose its efficacy. Suitable herbs to use in this way include ginger, fennel, lemon balm, chamomile, bitter orange, and helonias. Peppermint is an effective remedy for nausea and vomiting but is best avoided in regular doses during pregnancy; use catmint or spearmint instead, which are milder but just as effective. Similarly, although fennel is generally contraindicated in high doses during pregnancy, the few drops used in this approach are no more than would safely be used in cooking.

Infusions or decoctions of any of these herbs work just as well; ideally, prepare your brew and store in a thermos kept in the bedroom at night so that it is within reach before you get out of bed. Take regular sips of the mix throughout the day if required.

Ginger is, of course, ideal in a variety of forms: crystallized ginger or orange peel can be very tasty, or try ginger cookies or cakes, ginger ale, or ginger beer. Alternatively, take two 200 milligram capsules of powdered ginger three times daily.

If digestive problems are contributing to the morning sickness, take two 200 milligram capsules of slippery elm three times a day before meals or chew three to four slippery elm tablets before eating.

Sinusitis

Increased secretions from the nasal mucous membranes can lead to sinusitis, which is very common in pregnancy. Accompanying blocked nasal passages can lead to headaches if the sinuses (cavities in the bone structure of the face) become infected. There is generally pain between and around the eyes, which is usually worse when bending forward.

Simple anticatarrhal remedies, such as drinking elder flower tea (1 teaspoon per cup, three times a day) or using the chamomile inhalant suggested on page 25 can help. A little elder flower cream gently massaged into the painful areas around and between the eyes can also bring relief.

Sinusitis is often associated with an inability to cry and bottled-up emotions. If tension is contributing to the problem, then try some of the remedies suggested on pages 41 and 42.

Stress

Although, in theory, pregnancy should be a relaxed, blissful time for women, all too often it is quite the opposite—especially if the mother-to-be continues working full-time or is trying to cope with young toddlers.

It is important to allow plenty of time for relaxation: an hour a day for a leisurely bath and a breathing and exercise routine is important. If time is very tight, try to aim for at least thirty minutes a day. If you're working full-time, that rest period could perhaps be during the lunch break or immediately after you arrive home before family commitments intervene. No matter how busy your lifestyle, this pampering is important, so don't feel guilty that you're resting or concentrating on your breathing exercises while there are still chores to be done.

Herbs such as Siberian ginseng are ideal for increasing stamina and improving one's ability to cope with stress, but, as always in pregnancy, it is important not to take unnecessary medication. One 600 milligram capsule or tablet of Siberian ginseng daily for a fortnight should improve stamina and stress management. If need be, repeat the course after a two-week break, but try to avoid taking herbal tonic supplements continuously.

Other herbs that can help ease the symptoms of emotional stress are chamomile, hops, lemon balm, lime flowers, and skullcap. Use 1 teaspoon of any of these or 1 to 2 teaspoons of a mixture of two or more of them to a cup of tea and drink up to three times a day. Damiana infusion will also provide a tonic boost (1 teaspoon per cup per day), while eating oatmeal or taking oat extracts (1 teaspoon of wild oat tincture daily) can also act as a restorative for the nervous system.

The various Bach Flower Remedies or Californian Flower Quintessentials include many that are suitable for emotional or stress-related problems. Match your emotions to the remedies presented in Tables 3.1 and 3.2.

TABLE 3.1 *Bach Flower Remedies*

Remedy	Suggested Use
Elm	For feelings of inadequacy
Larch	For lack of confidence
Mimulus	For fear of known things
Olive	For complete exhaustion
Rock Rose	For panic or extreme fear
Scleranthus	For uncertainty and indecision
Sweet Chestnut	For extreme anguish; the limit of endurance
Walnut	Provides protection at times of change and during major life stage transitions, such as imminent motherhood
White Chestnut	For mental anguish and persistent nagging worries
Wild Oat	For uncertainty about which path to take; an aid to decision making

Stretch Marks

Stretch marks are caused by the skin suddenly stretching beyond its normal elasticity, which permanently damages the cellular structure. Stretch marks commonly occur across the abdomen and breasts and, while the initial bright-red striae will eventually fade, they never completely go away.

The aim is to prevent the marks appearing in the first place; to do this, it is essential to keep the skin well-oiled. Massage breasts, abdomen, and thighs (where the marks may also occur)

TABLE 3.2 *Californian Flower Quintessentials*

Remedy	Suggested Use
Alpine lily	For women who find it difficult to accept the physical nature of their femininity and are disturbed by the bodily changes of pregnancy
California pitcher plant	For those who feel weak or lacking in vitality
Dandelion	For those who try to cram too much into their lives, leaving no time for rest and relaxation; for overstriving
Dogwood	For physical tension and repressed emotions
Indian pink	For busy people who find it difficult to focus on the still center within
Lady's slipper	For those unable to draw on their inner wisdom and strength to provide energy for day-to-day needs
Madia	For those whose energy is easily dissipated; who feel distracted, dull, and listless
Mallow	For those who feel blocked emotionally
Pomegranate	For women finding it difficult to balance family and career demands
Quince	For women facing conflict between the nurturing role of a mother and the need to discipline their children objectively
Scotch broom	For those who feel depressed and weighted down about their lives
Yerba santa	For unresolved or repressed emotions, especially melancholy and grief

daily with suitable oils; the smell can be disguised with a few drops of lavender, neroli, or rose geranium essential oil if you find it unpleasant (add 20 drops of any of these essences to ¼ cup of wheat germ oil or olive oil and store in a suitable sterilized bottle. Vitamin E oil is also effective, or you can make a cold infused marigold oil and use that instead. You can vary the scents throughout your pregnancy. Massage is best after a warm (not hot) bath.

Teeth and Gum Problems

Yet another result of raised progesterone levels can be softened, bleeding gums. Regular visits to the dentist are essential to avoid unnecessary long-term damage. The old belief that women always lost teeth during pregnancy because of the calcium demands of the growing fetus really belongs in the realms of "old wives' tales." Teeth were lost because of poor general nutrition and softened gums; calcium is more likely to be leeched from the mother's bones than her teeth if there is any dietary deficiency.

Astringent and antiseptic herbs can be used as a regular mouthwash morning and evening. Use a well-strained, cooled infusion of agrimony, bistort, or lady's mantle or add 1 teaspoon of the tincture to a glass of water.

Vaginal Yeast Infection

Vaginal discharges often increase in pregnancy; this is due to the extended blood supply and congestion in the pelvic area as well as changes in the vagina's usual acid environment due to lower estrogen levels. These all provide an ideal breeding ground for yeast infections, such as *Candida albicans*, and the characteristic milky discharge soon follows, along with the associated soreness and itching.

Yeasts thrive in a warm, damp environment so try to wear loose cotton underwear and avoid nylon tights. Marigold cream can be applied to the vaginal area, or use a marigold infusion as a compress and apply to the vulva (the external area around the opening to the vagina). This can be repeated as often as necessary. Sitting in a sitz bath or a large tub containing chamomile or marigold infusion can also relieve symptoms. Instead of infusions, you can simply use warm water with 2 to 4 teaspoons of chamomile or marigold tincture or 5 to 10 drops of tea tree oil added.

Yeasts also thrive on sugar, so avoid sweet foods (including too much fruit sugar) and alcohol, and opt for showers rather than warm baths (which may also encourage the infection).

Internally, drink an infusion made from equal amounts of marigold petals and elder flowers (1 teaspoon of the mix per cup, three times daily) and take up to four 200 milligram capsules of echinacea daily. Garlic is also a good antifungal, so add some to cooking or use plenty of onions, if you prefer.

Varicose Veins

About one in ten women develop varicose veins during pregnancy. The muscle-relaxing effect of progesterone is partly to blame, along with weight gain, fluid retention, and pressure on the pelvic veins from the growing uterus, which all help limit the blood flow from the legs.

The problem worsens as the pregnancy continues, leading to heavy, aching legs with obviously distended veins in the later stages. The skin over the veins can itch, and there may also be swelling in the ankles and feet.

A simple remedy to tonify the veins is to shower alternately with very hot and very cold water for a total of five minutes each morning. Stand in the shower and hose your legs with cold water for as long as you can bear it, then switch to the hot tap and repeat. Alternate hot and cold for the rest of your five-minute session. Putting a brick under the foot of the bed at night will also help improve blood flow, but don't raise the foot of the bed if you are also suffering from heartburn or hiatal hernia.

Bathing the legs in diluted distilled witch hazel or witch hazel tincture can relieve the itching (one part witch hazel to four parts water; use distilled rose water or add a drop of rose oil if you prefer). Other useful herbs for external treatment include oak bark and horse chestnut; use the diluted tincture instead of witch hazel.

Internally, melilot and shepherd's purse tea (use equal amounts, 1 teaspoon of the mix per cup, three times daily) can help to improve venous blood flow and tonify the blood vessels.

4
More Serious Conditions of Pregnancy

Severe health problems in pregnancy generally need immediate treatment to prevent long-term damage to either mother or baby. Don't delay consulting your doctor if symptoms worsen or do not clear up after a few days. Have regular blood pressure and urine checks to identify potential problems before they become life threatening.

Ectopic Pregnancy

An ectopic pregnancy occurs when the fertilized egg latches onto the inner lining of the fallopian tube instead of attaching itself to the womb lining, or endometrium. Everything seems quite normal initially, but as the fetus starts to grow it causes increased pressure on the tube, with possible rupture and severe hemorrhaging.

Typically, around one in five thousand pregnancies is ectopic, so the condition is not that rare. Once a woman has suffered an ectopic pregnancy it is more likely to reoccur with subsequent pregnancies. The first sign is usually pain in the lower abdomen or to one side, which may be aggravated by motion and seem to radiate from vagina to leg.

Usually, but not always, the woman suspects she is pregnant and may have missed a period or had a positive pregnancy test. There may be a brown vaginal discharge or apparent bleeding, so it is easy to confuse the symptoms with a particularly painful period. Women may tolerate these symptoms for up to three weeks before seeking treatment. If untreated, the condition can be life threatening; the severe internal bleeding caused by rupture of the fallopian tube can be fatal. Hospital treatment and surgery to remove the mislocated ovum are essential.

Obviously, ectopic pregnancy is not a case to be addressed with self-administered herbs. More drastic measures are needed, but after surgery, Dr. Bach's Rescue Remedy or homeopathic arnica 6X will speed recovery. Herbal hormone regulators such as sage, lady's mantle, or chasteberry may be helpful to help restore normal menstrual activity once the woman has recovered fully from surgery.

High Blood Pressure

Weight gain, fluid imbalance, stress, and relaxation of blood vessels due to raised progesterone levels all contribute to the risk of high blood pressure in pregnancy. In some cases, hypertension is consistently present from the beginning of the pregnancy, but most problems start after the twenty-eighth week when the condition is sometimes called "gestational hypertension."

Although average figures for blood pressure are often based on age, everyone is different, and a "normal" blood pressure in pregnancy may be anything from around 110/70 to 140/90. Anything higher than this may restrict the blood supply to the placenta, which in turn may limit the baby's source of nutrients. High blood pressure can also indicate preeclampsia, which is potentially life threatening for both mother and child. Sudden and dramatic increases in blood pressure can occur in pregnancy, so regular checks are important.

For some women—especially if they have had blood pressure problems in a previous pregnancy—the very act of having their blood pressure measured is enough to send it racing upward. Opting for a home visit from a health care professional rather than the usual rushed trip to the doctor's office can often give a lower reading. Don't panic if an occasional measurement seems on the high side.

Simple dietary measures can often control mild cases; avoid stimulants such as black tea, coffee, cola drinks, spicy foods, alcohol, and cigarettes. Opt for a largely vegetarian diet with plenty of fruit, vegetables, legumes, nuts, and whole grains; limit salt intake and eat plenty of garlic (choose onions and leeks instead if you find that too much garlic leads to digestive upsets). Keep your intake of dairy products to a minimum and ensure a good mix of grains and legumes to give the right protein balance.

Drink 1 or 2 cups daily of an infusion made from equal amounts of hawthorn flowers and lime flowers; add an equal amount of dandelion leaves if there is fluid retention. Herbal medication is very effective at controlling blood pressure levels in mild cases, but because of the risks of preeclampsia or toxemia, it is vital to maintain regular contact with your doctor and, if necessary, take the orthodox medicines prescribed.

As always with hypertension, stress is a significant factor. Anxiety about other members of the family, fears of the birth itself, or concerns over the changing relationship with your partner can all contribute to the problem. Bach Flower Remedies, especially Mimulus and Rock Rose, can ease fears and anxiety. Adding 2 to 3 drops of lavender or rose geranium essential oil to the bathwater will also make a relaxing soak; or drink a cup of tea containing equal amounts of passion flower, chamomile, and skullcap once or twice a day as needed (1 teaspoon of the mix per cup).

Preeclampsia

Eclampsia is a potentially fatal condition associated with high blood pressure, swelling, and protein in the urine that can lead to convulsions and death of both mother and baby. It requires emergency medical treatment, and usually a Caesarean section is required. Preeclampsia, also known as metabolic toxemia, is the "buildup" stage when the condition can be treated and the pregnancy allowed to continue to term.

Research suggests that this problem may be associated with calcium deficiency and also the prior use of barrier contraceptives; others suspect poor nutrition and dietary deficiency, although the exact causes are still largely unknown.

It is definitely not a condition for home remedies, but herbs can be used to support professional management of the condition in consultation with your doctor or midwife. Regular cups of dandelion leaf infusion will act as a diuretic and also help maintain potassium levels; uva-ursi tea will also stimulate normal kidney function and increase urination.

Sufferers are generally advised to boost protein intake and include salt in the diet, since salt deficiency has also been associated with the condition. Orthodox practitioners generally prescribe potassium supplements and, apart from dandelion, other natural potassium sources include bananas, unpeeled potatoes, chicory, and uncooked beets.

Orthodox practitioners often prescribe a daily aspirin to women at risk for preeclampsia, although the research to support this practice is inconclusive. Herbal equivalents include meadowsweet and white willow (take a daily cup of either). Both, like aspirin, are rich in salicylates, which reduce platelet aggregation and stimulate the placental blood flow.

Symphysis Pubis Dysfunction (SPD)

The pubic joint to the front of the pelvis—the *symphysis pubis*—is also affected by the natural softening of tissues that accompanies pregnancy and widens to increase the diameter of the pelvis for the birth.

In some women, this widening leads to pain in the front pubic area that is worse when walking, spreading the legs, or lifting one leg. The pain may also travel to the groin and inner thighs. After the birth the condition generally resolves naturally and there is unlikely to be long-term damage, but the pain can be so severe that crutches are needed when walking. Your doctor may supply a support belt for daytime use and a tubular bandage to wear at night.

Minimize weight-bearing activity—including walking—and rest as much as possible. Try to keep your feet parallel when walking or even turn the toes in, pigeon style, to reduce any strain on the pubic joint. Go up stairs slowly and sideways, keep your knees together when sitting or getting in and out of the car, and avoid squatting. You can add a touch of glamour with a long decorative scarf tied around your hips. This will help reduce strain on the joint as well as demonstrate your fashion flair!

A warm bath with a few drops of lavender oil added may help relieve the discomfort; or apply a warm compress soaked in cramp bark decoction or lavender infusion. Homeopathic arnica 6x tablets taken three times a day for up to a week may also be beneficial.

Threatened Miscarriage

Miscarriage, especially in the first three months, can be nature's way of rejecting a malformed fetus. When it occurs in successive pregnancies, it may be related to the mother's health or uterine muscle weakness (which, in chronic cases, may require surgical intervention to ensure that the pregnancy goes to term).

Although a brown discharge or scanty bleeding each month can be quite normal during pregnancy, persistent or increased bleeding may indicate a threatened miscarriage. The usual orthodox treatment is bed rest until bleeding stops (a traditional approach that probably has very little effect on the outcome and can cause considerable strain to family life, especially if there are already young children in the house). Taking it easy for a few days will help, but threatened miscarriage really needs professional assistance.

Western herbalists usually prescribe a combination of false unicorn root and black haw. These herbs can help strengthen the uterus and also have a hormonal action. Use 1 teaspoon of the mix per cup as a decoction sipped every hour, or 5 drops of the combined tinctures in water. A cup of this mix daily during the first three months of pregnancy can also help women with a history of repeated miscarriage. Drink a cup of skullcap or chamomile tea to calm anxieties and encourage relaxation.

Chinese traditional medicine argues that miscarriage is related to weakness in the *Chong* (vital) and *Ren* (conception) meridians, and the classic formula to combat this is known as *Jiao Ai Tang*. Among other ingredients it contains *dong quai*, licorice, mugwort, and Chinese foxglove (*Rehmannia glutinosa*). It can be extremely effective but should only be used under the guidance of a health professional. I remember a patient whose first two pregnancies had largely been spent in bed because of persistent bleeding. With two small children, a self-employed husband, and a senile grandmother to care for, she could not face the same enforced rest a third time. *Jiao Ai Tang* taken for three weeks when bleeding started during the fourth month solved the problem and left the rest of her pregnancy trouble-free.

5
Childbirth

Modern Western medicine tends to make childbirth a high-tech affair with constant monitoring of the fetus, heavy dependence on painkilling drugs, and a medical fondness for Caesarean sections. In many states, midwifery services are limited, and home births with minimal intervention are virtually unknown. At the same time, many women believe that to "do their best for the baby" they must submit to whatever modern medicine demands of them.

For generations, herbal remedies were all women had to sustain them during a difficult labor or problematic birth. Given the high risk of death in childbirth endured by our grandmothers and great-grandmothers, no one would urge a return to such limited resources, but the herbs used are still effective and can certainly help during the early stages of labor and in the immediate postnatal period, when women are back at home and again able to take control and responsibility for their own health.

Preparing for Childbirth

While use of self-help remedies may be difficult during the actual birthing, herbs can be valuable in the final months of pregnancy to strengthen the womb and prepare the mother for the exertions to come.

There is a long list of traditional *partus praeparators* (preparations for childbirth). In Europe it includes raspberry leaf, lady's mantle, black horehound, motherwort, blessed thistle, and St. John's wort, while the herbs chosen by Native American women include squaw vine, blue cohosh, black cohosh, beth root, and false unicorn root. Some of these (notably false unicorn root and beth root) are really best left for professional use, as they are powerful stimulants.

Raspberry leaf is often the most readily available—sold in tablets and capsules as well as dried leaves for tea—and is excellent to strengthen the womb and increase pelvic flexibility for labor. Drink 2 cups of raspberry leaf tea every day during the last six weeks of pregnancy.

The other *praeparators* are just as effective: take 10 to 20 drops of blue cohosh, black cohosh, or squaw vine tincture in water each day during the final four weeks. Or use equal amounts of motherwort and St. John's wort in a daily infusion (1 teaspoon of the mix per cup) that will also help to calm the nerves.

Breech Babies

A breech birth occurs when the baby does not turn before delivery but presents with its head facing upward toward the mother's ribs rather than downward in the birth canal.

Many babies spend much of their time in the womb the "wrong way" up, but will turn naturally in the final weeks or even just before delivery. A breech birth can often progress quite normally with no more discomfort than a conventional delivery, although a skilled midwife will generally try to turn the baby, if possible, before birth.

If the baby is still in the breech position at thirty-four weeks, most women are advised to try a little intervention to persuade the newcomer to follow convention. Plenty of walking can help—the head is the heaviest part of the baby so will naturally drift downward under gravity when you are standing and moving around. If the baby is still the wrong way up during the final weeks, avoid squatting to try to prevent the breech engaging before the baby has turned.

Massaging the abdomen can also help. Ask your doctor or midwife which way the baby is most likely to turn (they will be able to feel its exact position and can tell you quite easily). Lie on the floor with your knees bent and your lower back resting on a pile of cushions so that your hips are higher than your head. Then gently massage your abdomen in the relevant clockwise or counterclockwise direction. Once you believe the baby has turned, stop all treatments.

During Labor

Labor can be quick and easy or it may take many hours, leading to exhaustion and anxiety. Prelabor contractions—a practice run for the real thing—can take place over several days. They are generally irregular and not as painful as true labor. This is usually preceded by a blood-stained discharge (the "show") as the mucus plug closing the cervix comes away, and a loss of waters when the amniotic fluid surrounding the baby is released. Labor should start within forty-eight hours of the waters breaking.

Once regular contractions are felt, the first stage of labor has started. Contractions start at around ten-minute intervals, gradually reducing over several hours to every two minutes; professional help is generally recommended from the five-minute stage. A long first stage may be due to insufficient contractions, leading to "uterine inertia." Weak, irregular contractions mean that the cervix dilates very slowly and labor is prolonged in a state of "hypotonic inertia." A simple way to encourage labor is sexual intercourse and nipple stimulation: both will increase production of prostaglandins and oxytocin, which are powerful hormones to activate the womb.

During this early stage, before orthodox medicine takes over, herbal infusions can help calm the nerves, stimulate the womb,

Herbal Birthing Kit

Planning your herbal birthing kit will depend very much on the approach of your doctor and hospital; if they have a positive attitude toward herbal medicine and are supportive, then your remedies can be used throughout labor and in the immediate postdelivery period. If they do not, your remedies will be confined to the home.

For Home Use in the Early Stages of Labor

- Herbal tea combination of equal amounts of wood betony, rose petals, squaw vine, and raspberry leaves. Use 2 teaspoons per cup, and sweeten with honey, if you wish. Drink as needed.

  OR

  Herbal tincture combination of 1 tablespoon of tincture of each of these same herbs mixed with an equal amount of water and stored in dropper bottles. Put 2 to 3 drops on the tongue as needed.

- If you are worried or apprehensive about the birth, mix 4 drops each of Dr. Bach's Mimulus, Hornbeam, and Rock Rose remedies in 1 tablespoon of spring water and store in a dropper bottle.

- For home massage of the lower back, abdomen, and inner thighs, put 10 drops each of lavender and jasmine essential oil in 2 tablespoons of almond or olive oil in a small bottle.

To Take to the Hospital

- A bottle containing well-diluted sage oil (10 drops per tablespoon of almond oil) for abdominal massage as labor progresses
- A thermos containing warm wood betony, rose petal, and mugwort tea with two or three cloves added, to help increase contractions during the later stages
- A thermos containing equal amounts of dried basil and motherwort tea to take immediately after the birth to help clear the placenta
- Arnica 6X tablets to take every fifteen to thirty minutes after the birth for a few hours to speed recovery
- A small bottle of infused marigold oil with 5 to 10 drops of lavender oil added to use to help perineal damage

For Home Use After the Birth (see chapter 6)

- 4 ounces of dried marigold or chamomile flowers to use in infusions for compresses and washes for perineal damage
- Dried raspberry leaf and fresh ginger root for use in treating afterpains
- A small bottle of black cohosh tincture
- Marigold cream for use on sore nipples
- 4 ounces of dried black haw or squaw vine or tincture for encouraging contraction of the uterus
- 4 ounces of dried lemon balm or St. John's wort or tincture to ease postnatal depression

and encourage the establishment of regular contractions. Start by sipping cups of tea made from equal amounts of wood betony, rose petals, squaw vine, and raspberry leaves, sweetened with honey if preferred. If drinking is difficult, mix tinctures of the herbs together, dilute 50/50 with water, and use drops of the mix on the tongue. It is obviously best to mix your dried herbs or prepare a tincture bottle in the days before labor starts. Wild yam (decoction or tincture) added to the mix can help relax the mother, especially if she is particularly nervous.

Bach Flower Remedies (such as Mimulus for fear) can also be helpful if the mother is nervous or anxious, while motherwort tea (2 teaspoons per cup) is a traditional remedy to calm anxious women during labor.

Massage is also helpful—your partner or a woman friend attending the birthing can massage your lower back, abdomen, and inner thighs using a mix of 10 drops each of lavender and jasmine essential oil to 2 tablespoons of almond or olive oil. Nutmeg and clove oils are also effective and especially popular in the East; use them in a similar dilution. Sage oil is another traditional remedy, although some women find it too stimulating, so start with 1 drop in 1 teaspoon of almond or olive oil and increase gradually to 5 drops if there is no adverse effect.

You can also apply a hot compress soaked in marigold, mugwort, or wood betony tea to the lower abdomen above the pubic area. Replace with another hot compress as it cools.

Weak and irregular contractions can be helped by drop doses of a combination of blue and black cohosh—dilute with water and use directly on the tongue every few minutes; alternatively, you can use diluted beth root tincture. All these herbs are powerful stimulants and should be used with caution, preferably with the guidance of a professional herbalist. Mugwort will also increase contractions; use it with wood betony as a tea and sip as often as possible. It is bitter tasting, so sweeten with honey if required.

By the end of the first stage, the cervix is nearly fully open and there may be a pause lasting from a few minutes to a couple of hours (the transition stage) before the second stage of labor begins.

The pattern of the contractions now changes to push the baby downward and out through the birth canal. This may take only a few minutes or several hours as the baby's head gradually emerges. This is when tears may occur if the perineum is not supple enough. In general, tears tend to heal better than cuts, so avoid a routine episiotomy (where an incision is made in the perineum before the head emerges) if at all possible.

The placenta will generally follow half an hour or so after the birth; its expulsion is stimulated if the baby is allowed to suckle at the breast as soon as routine examinations are complete. Modern orthodox practice generally includes injecting a medication to contract the uterus artificially at this stage, but mothers wanting a completely natural birth may prefer to discourage this standard procedure unless there is excessive bleeding. Putting the newly born baby to the breast before the cord is cut can help to expel the placenta naturally.

Herbs can be used to expel the placenta and stop bleeding. Many are extremely potent and really need skill to use effectively, and are best left to the professionals. It can also be difficult to take alternative remedies at this stage in the regulated environment of an American hospital. In Europe, herbalists and herbal medicine are increasingly acceptable to orthodox midwives, but in the United States this is not necessarily the case. One simple and gentle herbal option suitable for self-help is to drink a cup of basil and motherwort tea (1 teaspoon of each per cup) immediately after delivering the baby. Raspberry leaf tea can also be beneficial; or take a few drops of diluted shepherd's purse tincture on the tongue toward the end of the birth to help prevent postpartum hemorrhage.

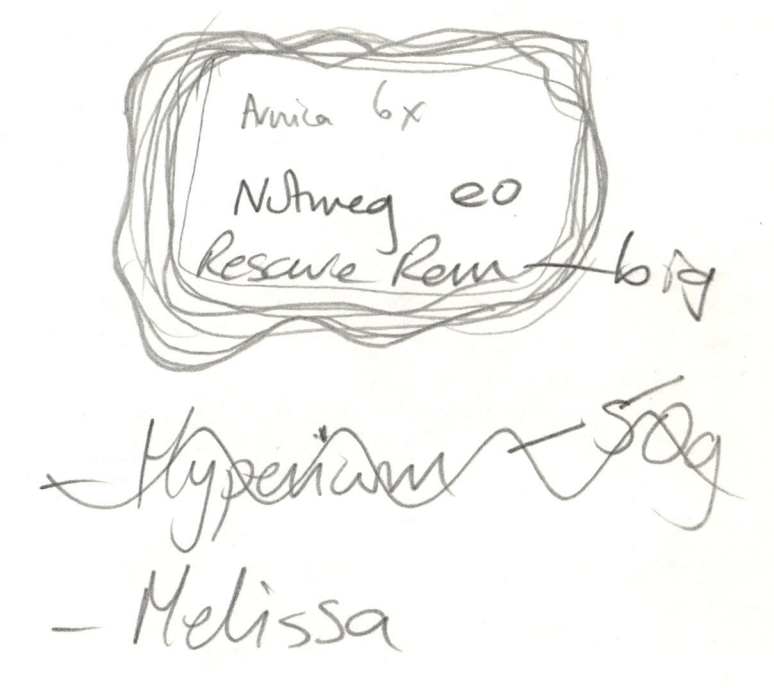

Immediately after the birth, start to take homeopathic arnica 6X tablets (one every fifteen to thirty minutes for several hours). These will help repair bruised and torn tissues and generally speed recovery from the shock of the birth.

[handwritten notes: Arnica 6x; Nutmeg eo; Rescue Rem — 6/7; Hypericum — 50g; — Melissa]

6
After the Birth

Today women are generally sent home within twenty-four hours of delivery unless there are complications or the patient is paying for private nursing. Many women prefer this approach; they can return to familiar surroundings and family life with their new babies as soon as possible. This is a far cry from my grandmother's day when a woman would not leave her bed for a month after the birth. Even during my mother's confinements in the 1950s, ten days in the hospital was still considered quite normal.

In theory, once back at home, the new mother should rest a great deal and have the support of relatives and friends when it comes to normal household chores. Unfortunately, many women, especially if they feel reasonably well or have older toddlers at home to care for, instantly return to the usual routine. A period of rest and taking things easy is essential. Not only is there a new young life to get to know, but childbirth can often be traumatic and exhausting, and it takes time to restore vital energies.

Postnatal care is important; birthing is a physical experience, and many parts of the body may have suffered bruising or damage. Any significant changes in the position of the womb and cervix should be noticed by doctors at the usual six-week medical check after the birth. There may also be bladder problems with increased frequency or possible leakage, at least in the early days. These will generally resolve without further intervention. Injury to the pelvic bones is not uncommon and an osteopath or chiropractor can often help restore alignment.

There are other changes to contend with as well. As hormone levels return to normal, many of the beneficial side effects disappear—that wonderful "bloom" of pregnancy fades and skin can become dry and scaly. Your baby may be demanding, but don't forget that skin cream and regular facials will once more be needed.

Afterpains

Cramping pains, particularly during breast-feeding, are common in the days following the birth as the uterus gradually contracts back to its prepregnancy shape. They tend to be more common with second and third babies than with a first birth but can be extremely uncomfortable.

A decoction of equal parts of black haw and wild yam (1 teaspoon of the mix per cup) taken three times a day will help to relax the womb and ease the discomfort. Raspberry leaf tea with a pinch of grated ginger can also help (again, drink 3 cups daily), or you can use 10 drops of black cohosh tincture in a little water.

Contraction of the Uterus

It can take about two months for the womb to return to normal after the birth. The process is helped by breast-feeding, which releases the hormone oxytocin into the bloodstream to improve lactation (that's why afterpains are common at feeding times).

Herbs can also help. A decoction or tincture of black haw (1 cup of tea or ½ teaspoon of tincture, three times a day) will help the womb return to normal; alternatively, drink 2 to 3 cups of squaw vine tea each day.

Perineum Problems

The perineum (the area between the anus and the vagina) is often cut during the birth as a routine procedure (episiotomy) or may have torn naturally. In either case, it is likely to be extremely sore and can take some time to heal.

Bathing the area frequently or sitting in a sitz bath or bidet can help: use 1 to 2 pints of infusion of lavender, marigold, St. John's wort, or comfrey leaves in the bath. If the area is not too sore to touch, then apply a cold compress soaked in these infusions (or distilled witch hazel) or soak a sanitary napkin in the same mix, freeze in the refrigerator, and wear the frozen pad until it thaws, replacing with another cold pad as necessary.

Creams can also help once the discomfort eases. They can be easily applied; use marigold or pilewort, which is astringent and healing and will help repair the damage.

Postnatal Depression

As progesterone levels fall back to normal, the sense of well-being and euphoria that the hormone brings fades and the "baby blues," starting on the third or fourth day after the birth, may begin. For many women this is simply a minor downturn when they feel especially emotional, may weep easily, and may experience irrational mood swings.

For a few women, this emotional time develops into a severe depression, which can persist for weeks or months. In severe cases, it requires hospitalization and lengthy separation from the new baby.

Adapting to a new baby takes time—especially with a first child—and can be especially traumatic for older mothers who are taking a career break and find the loss of work colleagues and stimulating conversation especially hard to bear.

While self-help herbal remedies are obviously inadequate for the most severe cases, they can certainly help with mild depression and ease the transition between lifestyles.

Lemon balm and vervain can be especially beneficial. Drink a tea containing 1 teaspoon of each, three times a day, or mix equal amounts of the tinctures and take 1 teaspoon in warm water. Borage and St. John's wort can also help. Again, use in teas or tinctures. St. John's wort is very widely prescribed in Germany for depression and is readily available in capsules and tablets that can be easy and convenient to take, especially when you're feeling down, preoccupied with a new baby, and with little spare energy to brew herbal teas.

Add a few drops of basil, rose, jasmine, neroli, melissa, or sandalwood essential oil to bathwater, or use the same oils in massage (2 to 5 drops of any of them to 1 teaspoon of almond oil).

The Shock of Parenthood

For many women, those first few weeks back at home with the new baby are a time of total chaos and confusion. These new mothers may feel permanently exhausted as the demanding new soul in their midst makes its presence very noisily felt.

Take your time with activities and try not to cram too much into each day. Many career women optimistically plan to return to work within weeks of the birth, but very few actually do. Not only do they find spending time with their babies intensely rewarding, but their mental confusion and exhaustion (not helped by sleepless nights) make normal work routines more difficult than usual.

The same confusion also affects fathers, who may also find their work routines adversely affected. If paid paternity leave is a possibility (as it is in many parts of Europe), it should certainly be taken.

Bach Flower Remedies can be useful for both parents trying to come to terms with the changes in their relationship and lifestyle. Walnut is ideal for times of change, while Rock Rose and Star of Bethlehem will help one cope with the overall shock. Many new parents spend the first few weeks in a complete daze, unable to relate to day-to-day events and finding it difficult to concentrate.

Soothing nervines, such as lemon balm and chamomile, make valuable teas for overexcited parents, soothing anxiety and tension, and liberal use of Dr. Bach's Rescue Remedy can also be helpful, especially in the early days.

The first weeks after the birth are a time for getting to know your baby and for your baby to become closer to you. Even though baby cannot understand your words, the sound of your voice is soothing, so be sure to chat happily to your baby during the day.

Encouraging your partner to take an active role in diaper changing and nighttime feeding also helps him become accustomed to the changing dynamics of the family. Many men quite happily undertake their share of nighttime duties, seeing it as a fair division of labor after the mother has spent an exhausting day caring for the new baby.

Tiredness

That month-long "lying in" period familiar to our grandmothers is for modern mothers little more than a few hours. Most women expect to be up and about within forty-eight hours after the birth or even sooner, unless there have been significant complications. Small wonder many women feel so tired.

Coping with the new routine of breast-feeding and sleepless nights is exhausting, and modern social pressures which suggest that women should be able to return to their prebaby routines as if nothing had happened do little to help.

Herbal tonics can help with tiredness: damiana and rosemary tea (equal amounts, 1 teaspoon per cup, two to three times daily) will provide a welcome energy boost, while eating oatmeal for breakfast also helps restore the nervous system. Raspberry leaf tea, ideally started before the birth, can easily be continued as a stimulating tonic afterward; it will also encourage milk flow.

A traditional Chinese tonic remedy for the mother to be taken in the weeks following the birth is to make a chicken soup flavored with a piece of *dong quai* and drink a bowl each day. Or add pieces of *dong quai* root to stews and casseroles; the flavor is not unpleasant. Capsules containing the dried herb are also available; take two 200 milligram capsules daily for at least six weeks.

Stillbirth

Losing a baby at birth is a traumatic experience from which some parents never fully recover. For the mother, there are all the physical signs of lactation, afterpains, and contractions on top of the emotional strain and grief felt by both parents.

Sage tea (1 teaspoon per cup, three times daily) will help to dry up any milk that has come in. Follow the recommendations given above to speed contraction of the uterus. Bach Flower Remedies—especially Sweet Chestnut and Gorse—can help with hopelessness and despondency. Many hospitals now accept the importance of allowing parents time alone with their dead baby as well as offering counseling services.

Try to take photographs (even a smudgy Polaroid is something to hang onto), name the child (ask for baptism if that is your belief), and hold a proper funeral or memorial service to give a focus to your grief. Allow yourself time to mourn.

7
Breast-Feeding

"Breast," as the enthusiasts put it, "is best." Breast milk is natural food for young babies and contains more than 200 important substances that stimulate and strengthen the baby's metabolism and immune system. It contains important trace elements, amino acids, and essential fatty acids not found in modified cow's milk formulations, and it is also a great deal easier to deliver than sterilized bottles and brewed powdered mixtures. But if for some reason you cannot cope with breast-feeding (perhaps you lack milk or have inverted or flat nipples that baby finds impossible to latch onto), don't feel that you are a failure. Feeding time can still be a positive experience with plenty of opportunity for cuddles and bonding, and you'll still be trying to do the best for your baby.

Preparing for Breast-Feeding

Breast milk is designed for babies, and there is no reason why breast-feeding should not be possible for most women. Ideally, the baby should be put to the breast on delivery, when its sucking will stimulate the production of colostrum—the rich, first milk full of important antibodies. Breast milk is easier for babies to digest than formula, and cow's milk fed to the very young can often lead to allergies and food intolerances in later life.

A good midwife will take the time to show the new mother how to help the baby latch onto the breast, sucking at the entire areola (the dark area around the nipple) rather than just holding onto the nipple itself. It is easier at first to take off your entire top and bra so there is nothing to obstruct baby's attempts to find the nipple. Nursing bras with discreet openings are ideal for public feeding once you have a little practice. Stroke the corner of the baby's mouth or cheek with your finger or nipple to trigger the characteristic "rooting" reflex that sends the baby in search of food. The sucking action will then stimulate milk flow.

It is important to adopt a relaxed, comfortable position before starting to nurse; a restless, irritated mother is likely to produce the same effect in her offspring. Sitting on a low chair with no arms but a good upright back support is ideal. Some mothers find sitting cross-legged on the floor with baby spread on their knees is more comfortable. Let the baby nurse on one breast for ten to fifteen minutes at each feeding time. After burping the baby or allowing him or her to take a short nap, break the suction by pushing your finger gently between the baby's jaws and then offer the other breast. If the baby is hungry she may drain this breast too. If not, she may just suck for comfort before falling asleep.

Breast-fed babies usually demand more frequent feeding than do bottle-fed babies; typically, the newborn may need to be fed ten times each day. This can gradually be reduced over six weeks to around six times a day. The usual pattern is three- to four-hour intervals between feedings during the day with the last one at 10:00 P.M., and then a single night feeding in the early hours. By four or five months, this is usually down to four feedings a day, plus some solid foods, with weaning beginning around six months.

Many herbs will stimulate milk flow, and drinking herbal teas while breast-feeding can be an effective way of giving the baby medication: agrimony tea drunk by the mother will ease baby's diarrhea, while chamomile will relax both mother and baby. Drinking regular cups of fennel, dill, caraway, or anise tea will not only help stimulate milk flow but also prevent baby's colic.

At the same time, remember that anything you consume may end up in breast milk, so avoid highly flavored foods (such as garlic and chili) as well as tea and coffee, which may overstimulate the baby. Orthodox medication taken during breast-feeding can also affect the baby, so be sure to tell your doctor that you are nursing when given any prescriptions.

Engorgement

Engorgement is most common in the first five days after the birth. The milk may come in suddenly in a rush, and be far in excess of the baby's needs. Expressing the milk with a hand pump can help; try increasing the frequency of nursing as well—small, frequent feedings can help keep the problem under control.

A warm compress soaked in lavender or chamomile tea will encourage milk flow when expressing the surplus. Less dramatic, but still annoying, is constant leaking, common in the early weeks. It is best to wear washable breast pads inside your bra to soak up any excess and use a little marigold cream on the nipples to prevent them from becoming sore from constant dampness.

Engorgement generally subsides quickly, although some women have a constant overabundance of milk and may need to express surplus milk throughout the breast-feeding period. Excessive milk production can be eased by drinking a cup of sage infusion once a day. This is also effective to dry up the milk at weaning time.

If engorgement is not resolved, mastitis (a painful inflammation caused when a milk duct becomes blocked and infected) may follow (see page 70).

Insufficient Milk

A poor milk supply may be related to inadequate nutrition, lack of rest, or stress, although some women are just naturally short of milk and find breast-feeding a problem in successive pregnancies. Large babies can prove very demanding, and it may be necessary to supplement feeding from an early age. Fashions change, but a few years ago it was common for doctors to recommend solids for larger babies at about six weeks of age.

Among the many herbs that have been used to encourage lactation are borage, fenugreek, goat's rue, milk thistle, stinging nettles, and vervain—as well as fennel, dill, caraway, or anise mentioned above and suitable for general use. Borage is available as a commercially prepared juice; take 2 teaspoons in water twice a day. Alternatively, you can use any of these herbs in teas (1 teaspoon per cup). Drink 3 cups daily, varying your choice to avoid becoming bored with any of the flavors.

Borage and vervain are also antidepressive, so choose them if you are feeling down.

Some of the hormonal herbs—notably chaste tree berries and saw palmetto—will also stimulate milk production; use tinctures and take 10 drops in water each day. Chaste tree will stimulate production of the hormone prolactin, which encourages milk flow, while saw palmetto has an effect on the mammary glands.

Mastitis

Mastitis (an inflammation of the breast tissue) can be very painful, with lumpy tender breasts and fever, and may require antibiotic treatment.

A traditional and effective remedy for mastitis is simply to insert a crushed cabbage leaf between bra and breast; replace every four hours. A poultice of fresh common plantain leaves is a good alternative to cabbage. Or use a compress soaked in hot water to which 2 to 3 drops of lavender, rose geranium, or fennel essential oil have been added; if you use these oils, make sure that the breast is wiped clean before nursing. A cup of tea containing equal amounts of red clover, chamomile, and marigold flowers (1 teaspoon of the mix per cup) taken three to four times a day will also help.

Sore and Cracked Nipples

Sore nipples are commonplace and generally caused by poor positioning of the baby, although they may also be due to sensitivity to the baby's sucking. Sore nipples are the most common reason for giving up breast-feeding.

One of the most popular remedies is marigold cream (often sold as calendula cream); in England many maternity hospitals now routinely give new mothers a tube of marigold cream when they are discharged. Apply to the areola after each nursing. Chamomile cream is also effective and can be used in the same way. Cracked nipples, often related to candidiasis, will also respond to marigold cream. If the baby has a yeast infection (see chapter 8), cracked nipples could easily become a persistent problem, unless the infection is completely cleared in the infant.

Other options include massaging the nipple with a little breast milk or buttermilk after nursing, or using 1 drop of rose or chamomile essential oil in 1 tablespoon of wheat germ oil to massage the nipple several times a day.

8

Easing Baby's Discomforts with Herbs

As every mother knows, each baby is totally unique and quite unlike any other. Some have a remarkably problem-free first few months of life—they sleep soundly, breast-feed easily, and suffer nothing more serious than occasional diaper rash. Others seem to cause concern from the start, with a constant series of minor health problems. If there are older toddlers in the house, the baby may go through his or her share of the usual childhood infections at a very young age. Try to keep infectious older children away from the new arrival to avoid too many demands on the immature immune system.

Colds

We all catch colds from time to time and babies are no exception, although the merest hint of a sniffle is often enough to send new parents into panic mode.

Early attention is, however, important. Babies obviously have very little distance between nose and lungs, so minor respiratory problems can easily develop into chest infections. It is important to avoid overuse of antibiotics, which can weaken the baby's immune system in the long run and are believed by some to contribute to the massive growth in childhood allergies seen in recent years.

Echinacea is an obvious choice for combating infections. Make a standard decoction of the root, dilute with an equal amount of water, and give the baby 2 to 4 drops with each feeding (dosage is related to body weight; for example, 20 drops daily for a 10-pound baby and up to 40 drops for a 20-pound baby). Elder flowers will ease congestion and are another safe remedy for even very young babies; make a standard infusion and give in drop doses at each feeding (use 1 drop per pound of body weight for each feeding). You can also soak a compress in warm elder flower and apply it to the baby's forehead while holding him to help cool fevers.

Similar drop doses of catmint infusion will also have a cooling effect on feverish conditions. Catmint is much gentler than spearmint, which can be used for older babies but can be irritating for very young ones. Spearmint is commonly grown as garden mint, so the fresh herb may be readily available. Use 1 teaspoon per cup for catmint infusions and ½ teaspoon if using spearmint.

If the baby has nasal congestion and early signs of a cold, put 1 to 2 drops of eucalyptus, tea tree, or lavender essential oil on a small piece of cloth pinned to the baby's clothing or directly onto the baby's mattress. The child can inhale the aromatic fumes and take this gentle antiseptic remedy directly to the seat of the infection.

Colic

Rushed or tense feeding times are often the cause of the gut spasms and discomfort of colic. Check the baby's diet (or your own, if breast-feeding) for possible irritants such as hot spices, cow's milk, or wheat and ensure that both mother and baby are relaxed and calm at mealtimes. Drinking a cup of chamomile or vervain tea between feedings will help.

Young babies will often accept herbal teas by bottle quite happily if they are started early enough. Recent studies in Great Britain demonstrated that babies will happily eat quite bitter-tasting vegetables at a young age, and introducing these foods early can prevent feeding problems at the toddler stage; it is the same with herbs. Catmint is ideal to soothe gut spasm and encourage sleep. Use 1 teaspoon of dried herb to 1 pint of water and give the baby 1 to 2 tablespoons of the warm infusion before meals. The surplus can be stored in the refrigerator for up to forty-eight hours and reheated before use. Dill, fennel, and caraway can be made into teas for the baby in the same way or be taken by the mother before breast-feeding.

Alternatively, make an infusion of chamomile flowers and use it to soak a compress to apply to the baby's abdomen to relieve colicky pains. Homeopathic chamomile (Chamomilla 3X) can be given in doses of 1 to 2 drops every fifteen minutes to relieve colic. It is also sold in pillules for older babies.

The Chinese massage part of the baby's lower back to ease gas and digestive upsets. Stroke the baby's spine from the lumbar region to the coccyx up to 200 times in one direction. If the baby is suffering from diarrhea, the motion should be from coccyx to lumbar area; stroke in the opposite direction to relieve constipation.

Cradle Cap

Cradle cap is scaly dermatitis affecting the scalps of newborn babies due to overactive sweat glands. It is not serious or contagious, although it does look unsightly and may cause new mothers to worry unnecessarily.

The traditional herbal treatment is heartsease; use the infusion as a wash to bathe the baby's scalp three or four times a day, taking great care with newborns whose fontanelles (soft spots) have yet to close completely. Marigold is also suitable if you do not have heartsease; the infused oils of either of these herbs can be used instead, if available. Marigold should be made as a cold infusion, and heartsease should be made using the hot infusion method. The oils can then be rubbed gently onto baby's scalp several times a day.

Diaper Rash

The red, painful irritation of diaper rash is very common and may sometimes be caused by irregular or inefficient changes and cleansing (for example, leaving the baby in damp soiled diapers longer than necessary). Mothers often blame diaper rash on their own shortcomings, but it can just as easily be related to digestive problems and yeast infections.

Regular diaper changes are obviously important, and it is essential to make sure the baby is completely dry before replacing the diaper—use a hair dryer on the cool setting if need be.

Use an infusion of heartsease as a soothing wash for the affected area before applying either comfrey or marigold oils or ointments. Ointments are better than creams in this case, as creams tend to blend into and soften the skin still further, while ointments will form a protective waterproof coating.

If there is any sign of infection, add 1 drop of tea tree oil to the heartsease wash before applying ointment.

Eye Problems

Sticky eyes with the eyelashes gummed together after sleep or pus in the corner of the eye are very common in babies and are usually caused by mild infections or, occasionally, a blocked tear duct.

Use a cotton ball soaked in a weak, well-strained infusion of marigold (½ teaspoon of dried herb to a cup of boiling water) to bathe the baby's eyes twice a day. A fresh, warm infusion is best, so make the mix as required and allow it to cool to body temperature before bathing the eye. Seek professional help if the condition continues for more than three days.

Conjunctivitis or pinkeye is also common and can be related to a vaginal bacteria infection in the mother. One to two drops of echinacea tincture at each feeding and bathing the eyelids with marigold infusion several times a day can help, but don't delay in seeking professional treatment if the condition does not clear up (as below) within three days.

Jaundice

Jaundice, characterized by a yellow tinge to the baby's skin and eyes, is common in newborns, especially if they are premature and have immature digestive systems. This sort of "physiological" jaundice can affect as many as three in four babies and generally clears up after feeding the first breast milk (thanks to the colostrum it contains).

Agrimony tea is ideal to help stimulate and normalize digestive function; drink 3 to 4 cups of a standard infusion each day, and the active constituents will pass into the breast milk to help your baby. Alternatively, you can give 1 to 2 drops of dandelion root decoction directly to the baby at each feeding.

Breast milk jaundice generally occurs after a couple of weeks. It is quite rare and is believed to be due to certain steroids in the milk affecting the baby's enzymes and preventing normal metabolism. As long as the baby remains well, the condition will generally resolve on its own after a few weeks, or you can switch to bottle feeding for a couple of days and see if the condition eases. Drink an infusion of equal amounts of agrimony and burdock leaves (1 teaspoon of each per cup) while breastfeeding to dose the baby or give 1 to 2 drops directly to the baby at each feeding.

Pathological jaundice, which may be due to congenital liver damage or disease, usually appears within the first week and is characterized by a lethargic and dehydrated baby. It needs immediate professional treatment if long-term effects, including brain damage, are to be avoided.

Unless you are confident that your baby has a minor, self-limiting type of jaundice, seek professional diagnosis in all cases.

Sleeplessness

Sleepless babies soon make the rest of the household tense and irritable, compounding the problem and leading to frayed tempers all around. Make sure the baby's room is not too hot and that he is comfortable and feels safe and secure—give lots of cuddles. Moving the crib to the parental bedroom or even taking the baby into bed with you is one solution, although parents who do this often find that it is a habit which is difficult to break and becomes a real problem as the baby moves to the toddler stage.

Young babies will often sleep more soundly if they are well wrapped in a baby blanket before bed. Tuck their arms inside the blanket and swaddle the baby with the shawl wrapped around the head and body, leaving the face exposed. This can be very comforting and reassuring and will also prevent overactive limbs from waking up the baby again as she is nodding off.

A chamomile bath is one of the simplest remedies for small babies; the herb is sedative and calming for the digestive system and is ideal to soothe overexcitement that can contribute to sleeplessness. Either add 1 cup of tea to the baby's bathwater or use 1 drop of chamomile oil (well dispersed in the water). Lavender infusion and oil can be used in the same way.

Older babies (beyond three months) can be give an infusion (1 to 2 tablespoons of tea made from 1 teaspoon of herb to 1 cup of water) at night using chamomile flowers, catmint, wood betony, or lemon balm.

Gentle massage can also help calm small babies; it is a traditional Chinese treatment for many ills. If the baby seems feverish and restless and is crying a lot and cannot sleep, try stroking her forearm repeatedly in one direction from wrist to elbow about 100 times. Repeat on the other arm. This part of the arm is called the "sky river water interval" in China and is associated with heat and feverishness. A little almond oil on your finger will provide lubrication and prevent irritating the baby's skin by the repeated motion.

Avoid caffeine-containing drinks (tea, coffee, cola) if breast-feeding, and check foods for artificial colors or additives that may lead to hyperactivity if the child is eating solids.

Teething

Teething usually is not a problem before four months, although it can start at a few weeks of age, adding to the stresses of coping with a new baby. A simple herbal option is to use the following gum rub to ease the discomfort.

Mix 2 drops each of chamomile, sage, and rosemary oils in 2 tablespoons of sunflower or almond oil and store in a clean bottle. Smear a small amount of the oil on your finger and gently rub the baby's gums with it; repeat three or four times a day as necessary.

Sedative herbs such as lime flowers or chamomile in weak infusions (1 teaspoon to a pint of water, given in tablespoon doses by bottle) can also help. Another option is homeopathic Chamomilla 3X pillules or drops.

A traditional Chinese remedy to ease teething pains is to put 1 drop of clove oil in a teaspoon of almond oil and use this to gently massage the baby's lower back.

Umbilical Care

The cut end of the umbilical cord is a potential site for infection, so it needs to be kept clean and dry with good air circulation. Make sure that diapers do not cover the umbilicus.

Traditional remedies for encouraging healing range from smearing the umbilicus stump with honey to simply applying a little distilled witch hazel. In most cases, as long as the wound is kept clean and dry it will heal quite naturally, but if you are concerned, bathe the area with a wash made by adding 1 teaspoon of echinacea tincture to ½ cup warm water. One to

2 drops of echinacea given internally can also be helpful if there are signs of infection. Slipping the drops into the baby's mouth as he sucks at the breast is often the easiest way to give the dose (or add to bottle feedings).

Yeast Infection

White plaques in the baby's mouth that do not rub off (unlike milk curds) usually indicate yeast infection from *Candida albicans*. The baby is likely to be restless and hungry, and the mother may have sore, cracked nipples as a result of the infection.

Mix 4 tablespoons of calendula tincture with 1 drop of tea tree and then add 2 to 3 drops of this mix to a small spray bottle containing a little warm water. Use this to gently spray inside the baby's mouth. Alternatively, use your finger or a cotton swab to gently apply this dilute mix directly to the affected area. Fresh aloe vera juice can be used instead, or smear the inside of the baby's mouth with plain yogurt that has live cultures, such as Stoneyfield Farm.

9
Herbs to Avoid During Pregnancy

Before taking any over-the-counter herbal remedy, remember to check contents against the list of plants to avoid in pregnancy, and note all individual cautions given for the herbs in the following sections carefully. Botanical names are included in the chart for those herbs not mentioned elsewhere in this book.

TABLE 9.1 *Plants to Completely Avoid During Pregnancy*

Name	Action / Cautions
Aloe vera	The leaves are strongly purgative and should not be taken internally.
Arbor vitae (*Thuja occidentalis*)	A uterine and menstrual stimulant that may damage the fetus.
Autumn crocus (*Colichicum autumnale*)	Can affect cell division and lead to fetal abnormalities.
Barberry (*Berberis vulgaris*)	Contains high levels of berberine, known to stimulate uterine contractions.
Basil oil	A uterine stimulant; use only in labor.
Beth root (*Trillium erectum*)	A uterine stimulant; use only in labor.

TABLE 9.1 *Continued.*

Name	Action / Cautions
Black cohosh (*Cimicifuga racemosus*)	May lead to premature contractions; avoid unless under professional guidance. Safe to use during childbirth.
Bloodroot (*Sanguinaria canadensis*)	A uterine stimulant that in quite small doses also causes vomiting.
Blue cohosh (*Caulophyllum thalictroides*)	A uterine stimulant to avoid unless under professional guidance. Safe to use during childbirth.
Broom (*Cytisus scoparius*)	Causes uterine contractions so should be avoided in pregnancy; in parts of Europe it is given after the birth to prevent blood loss.
Bugleweed (*Lycopus virginicus*)	Interferes with hormone production in the pituitary gland, so best avoided.
Clove oil	A uterine stimulant used only in labor.
Comfrey (*Symphytum officinale*)	Contains toxic chemicals that will cross placental barrier; do not take internally.
Cotton root (*Gossypium herbaceum*)	Uterine stimulant traditionally given to encourage contractions during a difficult labor, but rarely used medicinally today.
Devil's claw (*Harpagophytum procumbens*)	Uterine stimulant, oxytocic.

TABLE 9.1 *Continued.*

NAME	ACTION / CAUTIONS

Dong quai (*Angelica polymorpha* var. *sinensis*)
    Uterine and menstrual stimulant, best avoided during pregnancy; ideal after childbirth.

False unicorn root (*Chamaelirium luteum*)
    A hormonal stimulant to avoid unless under professional guidance.

Feverfew (*Tanacetum parthenium*)
    Uterine stimulant; may cause premature contractions.

Golden seal (*Hydrastis canadensis*)
    Uterine stimulant; may lead to premature contractions but safe during childbirth.

Greater celandine (*Chelidonium majus*)
    Uterine stimulant; may cause premature contractions.

Juniper and juniper oil (*Juniperus communis*)
    A uterine stimulant; use only in labor.

Lady's mantle (*Alchemilla xanthoclora*)
    A uterine stimulant; use only in labor.

Liferoot (*Senecio aureus*)
    A uterine stimulant containing toxic chemicals that will cross the placental barrier.

Mistletoe (*Viscum album*)
    A uterine stimulant containing toxic chemicals that may cross the placental barrier.

Mugwort (*Artemesia vulgaris*)
    A uterine stimulant that may also cause fetal abnormalities; avoid unless under professional guidance; also avoid when breast-feeding

TABLE 9.1 *Continued.*

NAME	ACTION / CAUTIONS
American pennyroyal (*Hedeoma pulegioides*)	Reputed uterine stimulant to be avoided in pregnancy.
European pennyroyal (*Mentha pulegium*)	A uterine stimulant that may also cause fetal abnormalities; avoid unless under professional guidance; also avoid when breast-feeding.
Peruvian bark (*Cinchona officinalis*)	Toxic; excess may cause blindness and coma; a specific for malaria and only given in pregnancy to malaria sufferers under professional guidance.
Pokeroot (*Phytolacca decandra*)	May cause fetal abnormalities.
Pseudoginseng (*Panax notoginseng*)	May cause fetal abnormalities.
Pulsatilla (*Anemone pulsatilla*)	Menstrual stimulant best avoided in pregnancy; limited use during lactation.
Rue (*Ruta graveolens*)	Uterine and menstrual stimulant; may cause premature contractions.
Sassafras (*Sassafras albidum*)	A uterine stimulant that may also cause fetal abnormalities.
Shepherd's purse (*Capsella bursa-pastoris*)	A uterine stimulant; use only in labor.
Southernwood (*Artemisia abrotanum*)	A uterine stimulant that may also cause fetal abnormalities; avoid unless under professional guidance; also avoid when breast-feeding.

TABLE 9.1 *Continued.*

NAME	ACTION / CAUTIONS

Squill (*Urginea maritima*)
    A uterine stimulant that may also cause fetal abnormalities.

Tansy (*Tanacetum vulgare*)
    A uterine stimulant that may also cause fetal abnormalities.

Wild yam (*Diascorea villosa*)
    A uterine stimulant to avoid unless under professional guidance; safe in labor.

Wormwood (*Artemisia absinthum*)
    A uterine stimulant that may also cause fetal abnormalities; avoid unless under professional guidance; also avoid when breast-feeding.

TABLE 9.2 *Plants to Use Only in Moderation During Pregnancy*

NAME	ACTION / CAUTIONS

Alder buckthorn (*Rhamnus frangula*)
    Strongly purgative, so should not be taken in high doses or for long periods.

Angelica (*Angelica archangelica*)
    A uterine stimulant in high doses, but quite safe as a culinary herb.

Anise and aniseed oil (*Pimpinella anisum*)
    A uterine stimulant in high doses, but quite safe as a culinary herb; avoid using the oil entirely.

Bitter orange (Citrus *aurantiam*)
    A uterine stimulant in high doses, but quite safe as a culinary herb or in moderate use.

TABLE 9.2 *Continued.*

NAME	ACTION / CAUTIONS
Caraway (*Carum carvi*)	A uterine stimulant in high doses, but quite safe as a culinary herb.
Cascara sagrada (*Rhamnus purshiana*)	Strongly purgative, so should not be taken in high doses or for long periods.
Celery seed and oil (*Apium graveolens*)	A uterine stimulant in high doses, but quite safe as a culinary herb.
Chamomile oil	The oil is a potent uterine stimulant to be avoided, but the dried or fresh herb is safe in moderation.
Chili (*Capsicum* spp)	Avoid high doses that may lead to heartburn and can flavor breast milk when breast-feeding; moderate culinary use is fine.
Cinnamon (*Cinnamomum zeylanicum*)	A uterine stimulant in high doses, but quite safe as a culinary herb; avoid the essential oil completely.
Cowslip (*Primula veris*)	Strongly purgative and a uterine stimulant in high doses.
Elder bark	Strongly purgative, so should not be taken in high doses or for long periods.
Fennel and fennel oil	A uterine stimulant in high doses, but quite safe as a culinary herb; avoid using the oil entirely.
Fenugreek (*Trigonella foenum-graecum*)	A uterine stimulant in high doses, but quite safe as a culinary herb or during labor.

TABLE 9.2 *Continued.*

Name	Action / Cautions
Garlic (*Allium sativa*)	Avoid high doses that may lead to heartburn and can flavor breast milk when breast-feeding. Moderate culinary use is fine.
Gotu kola (*Centella asiatica*)	Possible uterine stimulant; use in moderation for occasional teas only.
Jasmine oil	A uterine stimulant best reserved for childbirth to ease labor.
Korean ginseng (*Panax ginseng*)	Clinical reports suggest that high doses in pregnancy can lead to androgynous babies (caused by overstimulation of male sex hormones); use for short periods only.
Lavender (*Lavendula argustifolia*)	A uterine stimulant in high doses, but quite safe as a culinary herb or for moderate use.
Licorice (*Glycyrrhiza glabra*)	High doses can exacerbate high blood pressure; safe in moderation.
Lovage (*Levisticum officinale*)	A uterine stimulant traditionally used in slow and difficult labor; safe as a culinary herb.
Marjoram and marjoram oil (*Origanum vulgare*)	A uterine stimulant in high doses, but quite safe as a culinary herb; avoid using the oil entirely.
Motherwort (*Leonurus cardiaca*)	A uterine stimulant in high doses; best limited to the final weeks and during labor.
Myrrh (*Commiphora molmol*)	A uterine stimulant that may lead to premature contractions; avoid high doses.

TABLE 9.2 *Continued.*

Name	Action / Cautions
Nutmeg and Nutmeg Oil	Inhibits prostaglandin production and contains hallucinogens that may affect the fetus; once erroneously regarded as an abortifacient; safe in normal culinary use.
Oregano (*Origanum X marjoricum; O. onites*)	A uterine stimulant in high doses, but quite safe as a culinary herb; avoid using the oil entirely.
Parsley (*Petroselinum crispum*)	Uterine stimulant that may also irritate the fetus in high doses; safe in normal culinary use.
Passion flower (*Passiflora incarnata*)	A uterine stimulant in high doses; safe for moderate use.
Peppermint oil	A uterine stimulant; avoid the oil entirely, although low doses of the dried herb can be used.
Raspberry leaf (*Rubus idaeus*)	A uterine stimulant in high doses; best limited to the final six to eight weeks and during labor.
Rhubarb root (*Rheum palmatum*)	Strongly purgative, so should not be taken in high doses or for long periods.
Rosemary and rosemary oil	A uterine stimulant in high doses; safe in moderation and normal culinary use; avoid using the oil entirely.
Saffron (*Crocus sativa*)	A uterine stimulant in high doses; safe in normal culinary use.

TABLE 9.2 *Continued.*

NAME	ACTION / CAUTIONS

Sage and sage oil
: A uterine and hormonal stimulant in high doses, but quite safe as a culinary herb; contains thujone that may pass into breast milk, so avoid during lactation; avoid using the oil entirely.

Senna (*Senna alexandrina*)
: Strongly purgative, so should not be taken in high doses or for long periods.

Tea, black (*Camellia sinensis*)
: Limit to 2 cups a day, as excess can lead to palpitations and increased heart rate.

Thyme oil (*Thymus vulgaris*)
: Some reports claim that it acts as a uterine stimulant, although the research is disputed; the herb is quite safe in cooking.

Vervain (*Verbene officinalis*)
: A uterine stimulant in high doses; best limited to the final weeks and during labor.

White horehound (*Marrubium vulgare*)
: Reputed uterine stimulant; safe in moderation in cough drops.

Wood betony (*Stachys officinalis*)
: A uterine stimulant in high doses; best limited to the final weeks and during labor.

Yarrow (*Achillea millefolium*)
: A uterine stimulant in high doses; best limited to the final weeks and during labor.

10
Materia Medica

The herbs listed in this section are all featured in the specific remedies given earlier in the book. Some can be useful members of the home medicine chest at any time; others come into their own during the childbearing year. Some are typically "women's herbs" that are very specific for gynecological ills, such as chaste tree or blue cohosh. Other plants that have an important role in pregnancy and childbirth—wood betony, marigold, and St. John's wort, for example—have a far wider spectrum of use.

Few households will want to invest the time, space, or financial resources in assembling the entire collection of approximately one hundred different plants. A "top ten" to keep by you during pregnancy will obviously depend on your individual prevailing ailments and discomforts. Typically, the list might include

- American ginseng;
- bistort;
- butternut;
- chamomile;
- cleavers;
- ginger;
- lavender;
- raspberry leaf;
- slippery elm; and
- witch hazel.

For childbirth and the immediate postnatal period, helpful herbs might include

- arnica;
- basil;
- black haw;
- borage;
- fennel;
- lemon balm;
- rose;
- St. John's wort;
- wood betony; and
- vervain.

Whatever the choice, always be sure that the plant has been accurately labeled or identified before using fresh specimens, and buy dried herbs from reputable sources in small quantities to avoid deterioration. Take particular note of the plants to avoid in pregnancy, which are listed on pages 81–90. Many of these are potent uterine stimulants that can cause premature contractions; others contain toxins that can cross the placental barrier and damage the fetus.

Unless quantities are specified, the standard proportions given in chapter 11 should be used when making remedies.

Agrimony (*Agrimonia eupatoria*)

Agrimony is an astringent, bitter herb popular as a wound herb and digestive remedy. In the second century, Dioscorides used it for curing dysentery, and it was a major ingredient in fifteenth-century battlefield wound remedies. As a diuretic that contains silica, agrimony is also a good healing remedy for urinary disorders.

Parts used: aerial parts, leaves

Actions: astringent, diuretic, tissue healer, stops bleeding, stimulates bile flow, some antiviral activity reported

Uses in pregnancy: Agrimony can be helpful in a mouthwash for soft, bleeding gums and is also ideal taken as a tea while breastfeeding to treat mild diarrhea in small babies.

Aloe (*Aloe vera*)

Aloe is a tropical African plant that has been used since ancient times. In the West, the juice has traditionally been regarded as a soothing wound herb, although in Ayurvedic medicine it is considered a restorative tonic. "Aloe vera" is also the commercial name given to the mucilaginous gel popular both as a tonic remedy and as an ingredient in skin creams and cosmetic lotions.

Parts used: leaves, sap

Actions: antifungal, anthelmintic, bile stimulant, demulcent, purgative, styptic, sedative, tonic, wound healer

Uses in pregnancy: The fresh sap is healing for all sorts of scrapes, minor burns, eczema, and sunburn and is also suitable for oral thrush infections in young babies.

Caution: Use of aloe leaves as a purgative for constipation should be avoided in pregnancy.

American ginseng   (*Panax quinquefolius*)

American ginseng was discovered in the eighteenth century by Jesuits familiar with Korean ginseng from their missionary work in China who believed that a similar plant could be found in the remote mountains of North America. It is regarded as a gentler tonic than Korean ginseng, rather more *yin* in character and more suited for younger people and children.

Part used: root

Actions: adaptagen, aphrodisiac, digestive relaxant, lowers blood sugar

Uses in pregnancy: American ginseng is a gentler tonic in pregnancy than Korean ginseng and can combat fatigue and debility; it is helpful both before and after the birth. It is generally available in 600 milligram capsules of powdered root; up to 5 capsules can be taken daily.

Anise   (*Pimpinella anisum*)

Anise has been used as a spice since Egyptian times and is a popular flavoring for sweets and liqueurs. It is often used as a cough remedy, while the oil is used externally to combat lice and scabies.

Parts used: seeds, oil

Actions: carminative, expectorant, antispasmodic, mildly estrogenic, increases milk flow

Uses in pregnancy: Like its close relatives fennel and dill, anise eases indigestion, heartburn, and colic; it also helps stimulate milk flow when breast-feeding.

Arnica (*Arnica montana*)

Also known as leopard's bane, this daisylike alpine flower has a long history of use in central Europe as a remedy for bruises and sprains. It is still used in Germany for heart conditions, although internal use is restricted in many countries, as it is extremely toxic.

Part used: flowers

Actions: antibacterial, anti-inflammatory, astringent, bitter, heart stimulant, immune stimulant

Uses in pregnancy: Homeopathic arnica (6X) is used for shock, for traumatic injury, and to encourage healing after surgery; take it immediately after the birth to speed recovery. Arnica cream can also be used on painful varicose veins.

Caution: Because of its toxicity, arnica should never be used on broken skin and may cause contact dermatitis. It should only be taken internally in homeopathic doses.

Basil (*Ocimum basilicum*)

Familiar in Europe as a culinary herb, basil is regarded in India as a potent tonic, sacred to Vishnu and Krishna and capable of "opening the heart and mind." More prosaically, Western herbalism recommends it for digestive upsets, to clear intestinal parasites, and to improve digestion.

Parts used: leaves, essential oil

Actions: antidepressant, antiseptic, antispasmodic, stimulates the adrenal cortex, antiemetic, tonic, carminative, febrifuge, expectorant, increases milk flow

Uses in pregnancy: In the final stages of labor, basil has an uplifting, strengthening effect, as well as easing pains and helping to stimulate milk flow. The essential oil in baths or massage is helpful in postnatal depression, as is simply smelling the fresh plant.

Caution: Avoid the oil during pregnancy.

Beth root (*Trillium erectum*)

Beth root is a traditional Native American remedy to ease childbirth and treat irregular periods and other menstrual problems. It can reduce excessive menstrual bleeding caused by fibroids and is also used for bleeding associated with urinary problems. A douche is sometimes used for vaginal discharge and thrush.

Part used: rhizome

Actions: astringent, hemostatic, oxytocic, uterine tonic

Uses in pregnancy: Beth root is sometimes prescribed in the final stages of pregnancy to help prepare the womb for childbirth. It can also be useful as a decoction during labor to stimulate contractions.

Caution: Do not take during pregnancy unless under professional guidance. Safe to use during labor.

Bistort (*Polygonum bistorta*)

Bistort is believed to be the Saxon "atterlothe," one of the nine great healing herbs that the god Woden gave to the world. It is an extremely astringent plant largely used for bleeding—both internal and external—and for diarrhea. A little powdered root in the nostrils is a useful standby for nosebleeds.

Parts used: root, rhizome

Actions: astringent, antidiarrheal, anti-inflammatory, anticatarrhal, demulcent, styptic

Uses in pregnancy: A useful mouthwash for soft, bleeding gums that can also be used in compresses and ointments for hemorrhoids or perineal tears.

Bitter orange (*Citrus aurantium*)

The Seville orange—familiar from marmalade making—is also the source of a number of important medicinal products. The Chinese use both the unripe and ripe plants for indigestion and coughs. Neroli oil (see listing on page 123) is distilled from the orange blossom, bergamot oil, used for flavoring Earl Grey tea, from the peel, and petigrain oil from the leaves.

Parts used: fruit, peel, essential oil, flowers

Actions: antibacterial, anti-inflammatory, antifungal, aromatic, carminative

Uses in pregnancy: Take drops of bitter orange tincture or a decoction of the peel for morning sickness.

Black cohosh (*Cimicifuga racemosa*)

Black cohosh is a North American herb traditionally used to treat ailments as diverse as menstrual pain, whooping cough, and rheumatism. It is also popular in menopausal remedies.

Part used: root

Actions: sedative, anti-inflammatory, diuretic, combats coughs, menstrual stimulant, reduces blood pressure, lowers blood sugar levels

Uses in pregnancy: Black cohosh is traditionally taken in the last few weeks of pregnancy to prepare the womb for childbirth. It can help during labor to regulate contractions, and also to ease afterpains.

Caution: Excess can cause nausea and vomiting; the herb should be avoided until very late in pregnancy.

Black haw (*Viburnum prunifolium*)

Like its relative, cramp bark, black haw is primarily a relaxant useful as an antispasmodic to relieve cramping pains and also to calm the nerves. It is a specific for the uterus and will rapidly relieve menstrual cramps and related disorders.

Parts used: root bark, stem bark

Actions: antispasmodic, sedative, astringent, uterine relaxant, diuretic, lowers blood pressure

Uses in pregnancy: Black haw can help contraction of the womb after the birth and ease afterpains. Professional herbalists use the herb for threatened miscarriage.

Black horehound (*Ballota nigra*)

A straggling wayside plant often found growing in pavement cracks, black horehound was once used for dog bites and infected wounds. It was also popular for depression and menopausal problems, although there is little scientific evidence to support its action.

Parts used: aerial parts

Actions: antiemetic, antispasmodic, digestive relaxant, mild sedative

Uses in pregnancy: Black horehound is often recommended for morning sickness, but it does have a distinctive smell. Many women actually find that it makes them feel worse rather than better.

Black pepper (*Piper nigrum*)

Pepper originated in India but is now grown around the world. The various shades of peppercorns—white, green, red, and black—reflect different processing techniques. Black peppercorns are picked unripe and dried, whereas white ones are picked when ripe and soaked in water before drying. Black pepper produces an essential oil that is warming and very stimulating. It is used in aromatherapy for a wide range of ailments, including anemia and kidney problems.

Parts used: essential oil, seeds

Actions: antispasmodic, carminative, diuretic, stimulant, tonic

Uses in pregnancy: Black pepper oil is warming and soothing in massage rubs for backache and fatigue. It combines well with lavender or rosemary oils or can be added to bathwater. Only a very little is needed, so use sparingly.

Blessed thistle (*Cnicus benedictus*)

In the Middle Ages, holy thistle was believed to cure the plague and was widely used in lotions for "festering sores." Today it is mainly regarded as a digestive remedy, a bitter to stimulate gastric and gallbladder secretions. It is still also used in creams for wounds and sores.

Parts used: leaves, flowering tops

Actions: antibacterial, astringent, bitter, diaphoretic, expectorant, galactagogue, uterine stimulant

Uses in pregnancy: Blessed thistle is a traditional remedy to take during labor and childbirth to stimulate the womb and also encourage milk production. It is not as efficient a galactagogue as its relative, milk thistle, but is still worth using.

Caution: May cause vomiting in excessive doses.

Blue cohosh (*Caulophyllum thalictroides*)

Known as squaw root in North America because of its traditional role in treating various gynecological problems, blue cohosh is still largely used as a menstrual regulator and to ease uterine and ovarian pain.

Parts used: root, rhizome

Actions: anti-inflammatory, antispasmodic, uterine stimulant, diuretic, menstrual stimulant, antirheumatic, diaphoretic, uterine tonic

Uses in pregnancy: The herb is traditionally used in the final weeks of pregnancy to prepare for the birth; however, it needs to be used with care as too much may cause premature contractions. During the first stage of labor, it will stimulate and regulate contractions.

Caution: Avoid in pregnancy except during labor, unless under professional guidance, as it is a uterine stimulant.

Borage (*Borago officinalis*)

Borage stimulates the adrenal glands to produce adrenaline—the "flight or fight" hormone we make in moments of stress. It is also a sedative and antidepressant. Externally, the juice can be used to soothe itching skin, while the seeds are now known to contain gamma-linolenic acid—an essential fatty acid needed for various bodily functions.

Parts used: seed oil, leaves, flowers, juice

Actions: Leaves: adrenal stimulant, stimulates milk flow, diuretic, febrifuge, antirheumatic, diaphoretic, expectorant; *Juice:* antidepressant, topical antipruritic, demulcent, anti-inflammatory; *Seeds:* important source of essential fatty acids

Uses in pregnancy: Borage is one of the specifics for postnatal depression; it is uplifting for the nervous system while having a hormonal effect and stimulating milk flow.

Caution: Use is restricted in some countries, as it is related to comfrey and so contains traces of pyrrolizidine alkaloids.

Burdock *(Arctium lappa)*

Burdock root has long been used as a cleansing herb for skin and rheumatic problems or where a sluggish digestion is contributing to a buildup of toxins. In China the seeds are taken for feverish colds, and modern research does suggest some antimicrobial activity. It is a good source of minerals and vitamins.

Parts used: leaves, root, seeds

Actions: Root: cleansing, mild laxative, diuretic, diaphoretic, antirheumatic, antiseptic, antibiotic; *Leaves:* mild laxative, diuretic; *Seeds:* febrifuge, anti-inflammatory, antibacterial, hypoglycemic

Uses in pregnancy: One of the iron-rich plants that can be helpful for anemia.

Butternut *(Juglans cinerea)*

Butternut or white walnut is primarily used as a laxative. It has a gentler action than strong purgatives such as senna and cascara sagrada, so is safe to use in pregnancy. It is a cleansing remedy for skin problems related to an accumulation of toxins.

Part used: bark

Actions: anthelmintic, bile stimulant, hepatic, laxative, blood tonic

Uses in pregnancy: Butternut stimulates the digestion, so a decoction or tincture will ease constipation and can also reduce the straining that may lead to hemorrhoids.

Camphor (*Cinnamomum camphora*)

Camphor is popular in external liniments and rubs for muscular aches and pains and as a remedy for chilblains. In Ayurvedic medicine the herb is believed to open the senses and bring clarity. It is only used externally in the Western tradition, although in India the crystals are used as snuff for nasal congestion and other ailments.

Parts used: a crystalline extract made from the wood and leaves

Actions: bitter, stimulant for the circulation and nervous system, anti-inflammatory, analgesic, antispasmodic, antiparasitic

Uses in pregnancy: Camphor has a pungent, stimulating smell that can be sniffed to combat feelings of faintness; use a little camphorated oil or lotion on a handkerchief and inhale the fumes. Traditional smelling-salt bottles contained a cotton swab soaked in camphor. Externally, camphorated oil can be useful as a warming rub for both backache and chilblains.

Caution: Do not take internally.

Caraway (*Carum carvi*)

Caraway seed is widely used in Middle Eastern dishes and for flavoring breads and cakes. Like many culinary herbs, it has a calming effect on the digestion and is mainly used for stomach complaints or to relieve menstrual cramps.

Parts used: oil, seeds

Actions: antimicrobial, antispasmodic, carminative, emmenagogue, expectorant, stimulates milk flow

Uses in pregnancy: Caraway is included in remedies for gas and colic in babies. As it also stimulates milk flow, nursing mothers can improve lactation and combat baby's digestive upsets by drinking regular infusions.

Caution: Avoid high doses during pregnancy, as it is a uterine stimulant.

Catmint *(Nepeta cataria)*

Catmint, as the name suggests, is a favorite with cats who will roll in ecstasy in a bed of the plant. It is a gentle herb ideal for children and suitable for colic, feverish chills, and hyperactivity. Like other members of the mint family it will also ease the symptoms of indigestion and nausea, but, unlike peppermint, it does not contain the irritant menthol.

Parts used: aerial parts

Actions: antispasmodic, diaphoretic, carminative, gentle nerve relaxant, antidiarrheal, increases menstrual flow

Uses in pregnancy: A gentle remedy for morning sickness; also suitable for colic and gas in small babies.

Chamomile *(Matricaria recutita/ Chamaemelum nobile)*

Both German chamomile (*M. recutita*) and its relative Roman chamomile (*C. nobile*) are among the most widely used of medicinal herbs. Their actions are very similar, with Roman chamomile having a slightly more bitter taste and German chamomile rather more anti-inflammatory, antiseptic, and analgesic. The Greeks called the herb "ground apple" (*kamai melon*) because of its characteristic smell.

Parts used: flowers, essential oil

Actions: antiemetic, anti-inflammatory, antispasmodic, antimicrobial, antiseptic, bitter, carminative, mild anodyne, sedative

Uses in pregnancy: As an antiemetic, chamomile can be helpful for morning sickness while its sedative properties are ideal for stress-related hypertension, anxiety, and insomnia. Externally, a cream is soothing for skin infections and inflammations, including thrush, diaper rash, hemorrhoids, and sore nipples. It is also gentle enough for babies suffering from sleeplessness, colic, and teething (ideally as homeopathic Chamomilla 3X). The oil, although expensive, can be used sparingly in massage rubs for backaches and nerve pains.

Chaste tree (*Vitex agnus-castus*)

The chaste tree reputedly takes its name from its action as a male anaphrodisiac, used by medieval monks to reduce libido. It acts on the pituitary gland to increase the production of female sex hormones involved in ovulation, so it is extremely useful in numerous gynecological conditions.

Part used: berries

Actions: Pituitary stimulant and hormone regulator, reproductive tonic, increases milk production, female aphrodisiac, male anaphrodisiac

Uses in pregnancy: The herb can help to normalize and stimulate the menstrual cycle before conception to combat female infertility. It is helpful for breast-feeding when there is poor milk production related to hormonal problems.

Caution: Excess can create the sensation of ants crawling over the skin.

Cleavers (*Galium aparine*)

Usually dismissed as a weed, cleavers is an important lymphatic cleanser once used to feed domestic geese; hence its country name, "goosegrass."

Parts used: aerial parts

Actions: diuretic, lymphatic cleanser, mild astringent

Uses in pregnancy: The fresh herb is especially diuretic and can be helpful for fluid retention and edema.

Cloves (*Syzygium aromaticum*)

Cloves have been used for flavoring for around 2,000 years and were known in Roman times as an exotic spice. The Chinese consider the plant a kidney tonic, increasing *yang* energy and ideal for treating male impotence.

Parts used: flower buds, essential oil

Actions: mild anesthetic, anodyne, antiemetic, antiseptic, antispasmodic, carminative, warming stimulant

Uses in pregnancy: In many parts of the East, clove oil is used for abdominal massage during labor to encourage contractions and ease discomfort. Drinking teas flavored with plenty of cloves during the second stage of labor can help to ease childbirth pains.

Caution: Cloves should be reserved for labor and childbirth and not taken earlier in pregnancy.

Comfrey (*Symphytum officinale*)

Comfrey has been used for centuries as a wound healer and restorer of broken bones; it was once known as "knitbone," while the botanical name is derived from the Greek *sympho*, meaning "to unite." Its healing action is due to a chemical called allantoin, which encourages cell growth to accelerate healing.

Parts used: root, leaves

Actions: astringent, cell proliferant, demulcent, expectorant, wound herb

Uses in pregnancy: Comfrey is ideal externally for any sort of tissue damage; it can be especially helpful for perineal tears or severe diaper rash.

Caution: During the 1960s and 1970s the plant became over-hyped as a cure-all for arthritis. In animal studies the plant was blamed for causing liver tumors due to its high pyrrolizidine alkaloid content. Its use has since been banned in many countries, although many consider its risks greatly overemphasized (Betz et al. 1994). It should not be used on fresh wounds before they are thoroughly cleaned since the rapid healing caused by the allantoin may trap dirt, leading to abscesses. Because of these concerns some mothers may be reluctant to use the herb for treating diaper rash, one of its traditional applications.

Couch grass (*Elymus repens*)

Regarded by gardeners as an invasive weed, couch grass is valued by herbalists as a soothing remedy for cystitis, prostate problems, and kidney infections, and is also added to remedies for gout and rheumatism.

Part used: rhizome

Actions: diuretic, emollient, laxative, urinary antiseptic

Uses in pregnancy: Couch grass is ideal for cystitis and fluid retention. It can be used in decoctions, and the dried herb is also sold in capsules.

Cornsilk (*Zea mays*)

Cornsilk begins as the long, silky stamens from corn plants which dry to form a crinkled mass resembling red beard clippings. It is a soothing diuretic for an irritated and inflamed bladder and urinary tract disorders, including prostate problems.

Part used: stamens

Actions: diuretic, soothing for the urinary tract, mild bile stimulant

Uses in pregnancy: The herb is helpful for fluid retention and cystitis; it can also reduce bed-wetting in small children when this is associated with bladder irritation.

Cramp bark (*Viburnum opulus*)

Cramp bark, as the name suggests, is a useful relaxant for both muscles and nerves. It can ease the spasms of cramp and colic and will combat constipation, especially when related to tension and anxiety. It will also relax the blood vessels to reduce high blood pressure. Externally, it can be used in creams and lotions to relieve muscle cramps.

Part used: bark

Actions: antispasmodic, sedative, astringent, muscle relaxant, nervine

Uses in pregnancy: Cramp bark decoction can be safely used to lower high blood pressure in mild cases, although its main benefit in pregnancy is to ease muscular cramps.

Cranberry (*Vitis macrocarpon*)

Cranberries, a North American fruit, were used by Native Americans in wound dressings and were first cultivated in New England in 1816. Medical interest in the plant has revived in recent years following studies that demonstrated its efficacy in treating cystitis. The herb is closely related to uva-ursi, an important urinary antiseptic.

Parts used: leaves, berries

Actions: antibacterial, antiseptic, antiemetic, astringent, hypoglycemic, tonic, high vitamin C content

Uses in pregnancy: Externally, the berries can be used in creams and ointments for hemorrhoids and minor wounds, while the juice is ideal as a preventive for urinary infections for those prone to recurrent cystitis.

Damiana (*Turnera diffusa* var. *aphrodisiaca*)

Damiana is a popular aphrodisiac from Central America. It acts as a tonic for the nervous system and as an antidepressant but is also stimulating for the digestion and urinary system, useful in convalescence, and for general debility. Although largely regarded as a potent male aphrodisiac because of its testosterogenic action, it can be helpful for various gynecological disorders as well.

Part used: leaves

Actions: stimulant, tonic, antidepressant, laxative, diuretic, aphrodisiac, testosterogenic

Uses in pregnancy: Damiana can be helpful for male infertility or loss of libido affecting conception. After the birth it makes a useful tonic herb for new mothers taken as a daily tea; it can also be used for those prone to low blood pressure and fainting.

Dandelion (*Taraxacum officinale*)

Dandelion is a comparative newcomer to Western herbalism, first mentioned in the fifteenth century. The plant is strongly diuretic, so it is often used for fluid retention and urinary problems. The root is also very cleansing for the liver and a mild laxative; it is often used in chronic skin problems and arthritis.

Parts used: leaves, root

Actions: Leaves: diuretic, hepatic and digestive tonic; *Root:* liver tonic, stimulates bile flow, diuretic, laxative, antirheumatic

Uses in pregnancy: As an effective diuretic, dandelion can be helpful for edema or fluid retention and is used with other herbs to combat preeclampsia. The leaves are very rich in minerals (valuable in anemia), while the root is a gentle laxative suitable for constipation during pregnancy.

Dill (*Anethum graveolens*)

Dill is carminative and soothing for the stomach and is an ideal remedy for baby's colic and gas. The seeds can be chewed to relieve bad breath, and it can also help with menstrual cramps.

Parts used: seeds, essential oil, leaves

Actions: carminative, antispasmodic, increases milk production

Uses in pregnancy: Dill tea will help to stimulate milk production in nursing mothers, while the same mix will help with baby's digestion. Dill is the prime ingredient in baby's "gripe water," a traditional remedy for easing colic.

Dong quai / Chinese angelica (*Angelica polymorpha* var. *sinensis*)

In China, *dong quai* is regarded as the most important tonic herb after ginseng. It is used as a blood tonic for anemia, menstrual problems, or after childbirth and is also a mild laxative especially suitable for the elderly. It is sometimes sold as "tang kwai" in the West (using an older system of Chinese transliteration).

Parts used: rhizome

Actions: blood tonic, circulatory stimulant, laxative, antispasmodic, some antibacterial action

Uses in pregnancy: Dong quai is a valuable gynecological tonic in infertility and also after childbirth when it is traditionally cooked in chicken soup to make a highly nutritious food. It is an ingredient of *Jiao Ai Tang*, a traditional Chinese remedy for threatened miscarriage.

Caution: Dong quai should be avoided in pregnancy except with professional guidance.

Echinacea   (*Echinacea angustifolia, E. pallida, E. purpurea*)

Echinacea, or purple cone flower, was one of the most important herbs used by Native American healers, who regarded it as something of a cure-all. Interest in the plant spread to Europe in the 1930s when research in Germany highlighted its potent antibiotic actions.

Parts used: root, aerial parts

Actions: antibiotic, antiallergenic, anti-inflammatory, immune stimulant, lymphatic tonic, wound herb

Uses in pregnancy: Echinacea is a valuable alternative to orthodox antibiotics for infections in pregnancy. It is a specific for urinary infections which, if chronic, may also be contributing to infertility.

Elder   (*Sambucus nigra*)

The elder has long been regarded as a complete medicine chest: the leaves form the basis of a "green ointment" for sprains and strains; the inner bark is a strong purgative; the berries, a good source of vitamin C, act as a prophylactic against colds and infections; and the flowers are strongly anticatarrhal.

Parts used: Collect the flowers in spring, the leaves in summer after flowering, and the berries in autumn. The bark, leaves, and roots have all been used in the past.

Actions: anti-inflammatory, anticatarrhal, diaphoretic, diuretic, emollient (flowers), laxative (berries and bark)

Uses in pregnancy: Elder flower cream can be helpful for skin inflammations and sores and works well, combined with calendula, for thrush and other fungal infections. Use the infusion for catarrhal problems or infections. If you have no dried elder flowers for your tea, use a teaspoon of concentrated elder flower cordial diluted with hot water instead. The cream also makes a useful massage rub to ease blocked and infected sinuses.

False unicorn root/ Helonias *(Chamaelirium luteum)*

Another of the traditional Native American herbs, false unicorn root was used by tribes in Arkansas for treating ulcers, diarrhea, and urinary problems. It is mainly used in the West for gynecological disorders, including ovarian cysts and menopausal difficulties.

Part used: root

Actions: uterine and ovarian tonic, menstrual stimulant, diuretic, estrogenic, bitter

Uses in pregnancy: False unicorn root can be helpful to regulate and stimulate menstrual function before conception to improve fertility. Drops of the tincture can also be useful to counter morning sickness. The plant is used by professional herbalists to combat threatened miscarriage and also as a traditional *partus praeparator*, taken in the weeks before the birth to strengthen the uterus.

Caution: False unicorn root is a potent herb and is best used under professional guidance in pregnancy.

Fennel *(Foeniculum officinalis)*

Fennel has been cultivated as a vegetable since Roman times; the Greeks called it *marathron*, derived from a verb meaning "to grow thin," and seem to have considered it an early slimming aid.

Parts used: seeds; stem base eaten as a vegetable

Actions: anti-inflammatory, carminative, circulatory stimulant, diuretic, mild expectorant, stimulates milk production

Uses in pregnancy: Like its close relative, dill, fennel seed tea is ideal for indigestion, gas, or colic and is a regular component in baby's "gripe water." Drops of the tincture can help regulate the digestion to combat morning sickness, while the tea will stimulate milk production in nursing mothers.

Fenugreek   (*Trigonella foenum-graecum*)

The potent aroma and taste of fenugreek are familiar in Indian and Middle Eastern cookery, and the herb gives a spicy flavor to curries, pickles, and garnishes. The seeds are mainly used in herbal medicine as a warming remedy for stomach and kidney chills, while the whole dried plant is used in modern Egypt for spasmodic abdominal pain.

Parts used: seeds, whole herb

Actions: anti-inflammatory, digestive tonic, stimulates milk production, locally demulcent, uterine stimulant, hypoglycemic

Uses in pregnancy: Fenugreek is ideal after the birth to stimulate milk production, although too much may give breast milk a spicy flavor!

Caution: Avoid during pregnancy as it is a uterine stimulant. Insulin-dependent diabetics should not take the plant without professional advice.

Garlic   (*Allium sativa*)

Garlic has been used as a medicinal herb for at least 5,000 years. Its characteristic smell is due to a group of sulphur-containing compounds, notably allicin, which account for its medicinal activity.

Part used: clove

Actions: antibiotic, antihistamine, antiparasitic, antithrombotic, diaphoretic, expectorant, hypotensive, reduces cholesterol levels, reduces blood sugar levels

Uses in pregnancy: Garlic can be used in pregnancy for treating vaginal yeast infection, which may also be contributing to infertility if conception is a problem. In low doses, it's a useful supplement to help prevent infection and stimulate digestive function.

Caution: High doses of garlic are best avoided in pregnancy and breast-feeding as they may lead to heartburn or flavor breast milk.

Ginger (*Zingiber officinalis*)

Ginger is listed in some of the earliest Chinese herbals and has been used in warming decoctions for stomach upsets, colds, and chills since Roman times. It is one of our best antiemetics and has been successfully used in clinical trials in cases of very severe morning sickness.

Parts used: root, essential oil

Actions: antiemetic, antiseptic, antispasmodic, carminative, circulatory stimulant, diaphoretic, expectorant, peripheral vasodilator; topically as a rubefacient

Uses in pregnancy: Ginger is best taken in tinctures, decoctions, capsules, or, perhaps more pleasantly, as crystallized ginger sweets or in ginger beer and biscuits for morning sickness. The essential oil used in massage rubs will encourage blood flow to ease muscular stiffness, aches, and pains. A pinch of grated ginger, or a drop of the oil, can be added to infusions and decoctions to ease afterpains.

Ginseng (*Panax ginseng*)

Ginseng has been used in China for more than 5,000 years and is believed to strengthen the body's vital energy (*qi*). The plant is rich in steroidal compounds that are very similar to human sex hormones; hence its reputation as an aphrodisiac, although it also acts as an all-around tonic, helping the body adapt to stressful situations.

Part used: root

Actions: tonic, stimulant, reduces blood sugar and cholesterol levels, immunostimulant

Uses in pregnancy: Ginseng can help with male infertility problems and is an ideal tonic for both partners after birth if fatigue and debility are problems. A daily ginseng capsule to combat low blood pressure and fainting spells may also be useful for short-term use.

Caution: Do not take for more than four weeks without a break; avoid taking with caffeine and during pregnancy.

Goat's rue (*Galega officinalis*)

Once a favorite treatment for plague, goat's rue is now largely used in late-onset diabetes to normalize blood sugar levels. It will reputedly increase breast size.

Part used: leaves

Actions: antidiabetic, lowers blood sugar levels, diuretic, diaphoretic, increases milk flow

Uses in pregnancy: Drinking goat's rue tea is one of the most effective ways to stimulate milk flow during breast-feeding.

Caution: Should not be taken by insulin-dependent diabetics without professional supervision.

Hawthorn (*Crataegus laevigata, C. monogyna*)

Hawthorn is widely used as a cardiac tonic and will improve peripheral circulation, regulate heart rate and blood pressure, and improve coronary blood flow.

Parts used: flowering tops, berries

Actions: cardiotonic, vasodilator, relaxant, antispasmodic, regulates blood pressure, diuretic

Uses in pregnancy: Hawthorn is one of the herbs that can safely be used in pregnancy to reduce high blood pressure; it works well with lime flowers and makes a pleasant tea. The berries will also help ease cramps. Because it normalizes blood pressure levels, it can also be useful if low blood pressure and fainting are problems.

Heartsease (*Viola tricolor*)

Heartsease, or wild pansy, is a popular garden flower that is good for coughs, bronchitis, and whooping cough and soothes skin inflammations and eczema. It is rich in flavonoids (including rutin), so it will strengthen capillary walls.

Parts used: aerial parts

Actions: expectorant, anti-inflammatory, diuretic, antirheumatic, laxative, stabilizes capillary membranes

Uses in pregnancy: Heartsease infusion can be used in creams or as a wash to bathe skin sores, diaper rash, and cradle cap.

Horsetail (*Equisetum arvense*)

Horsetails grew in prehistoric times, and their decayed remains form much of the world's coal seams. The plant is rich in silica, which is very healing, and is used for urinary tract problems, including prostate disorders, as well as for deep-seated lung problems, including chronic bronchitis.

Parts used: aerial parts

Actions: astringent, styptic, diuretic, anti-inflammatory, tissue healer

Uses in pregnancy: As a diuretic, horsetail can be helpful in fluid retention and bladder inflammations. Apart from silica, the plant also contains calcium and potassium salts, so it is a useful mineral source to combat cramps.

Horse chestnut *(Aesculus hippocastanum)*

Horse chestnut extracts are largely used for rheumatism, hemorrhoids, and varicose veins. The main active component is aescin, an anti-inflammatory saponin that is sometimes extracted for use in over-the-counter products. It can be used internally and externally.

Parts used: bark, seeds

Actions: anti-inflammatory, antiedema, astringent, tonifies and relaxes blood vessels

Uses in pregnancy: Drink a decoction or use it as a wash for hemorrhoids, varicose veins, and swollen ankles. Commercial creams or gels can be used externally instead.

Ispaghula/Psyllium *(Plantago psyllium, P. ovata)*

Ispaghula seeds swell when moistened to form a glutinous mass that encourages peristalsis and lubricates the bowel. Although primarily used for constipation, the resulting bulky mass can help to soothe diarrhea and is also recommended for irritable bowel syndrome.

Parts used: seeds, husks

Actions: demulcent, bulk laxative, antidiarrheal

Uses in pregnancy: Ideal for constipation and to reduce straining, which may lead to hemorrhoids.

Caution: Always take capsules or dried psyllium with plenty of water.

Jasmine (*Jasminium officinale*)

The heavy scent of jasmine makes it a favorite garden flower and a popular oil in perfumery. It is used in aromatherapy as an antidepressant and antispasmodic massage for menstrual pains. It is an effective aphrodisiac for both men and women.

Part used: essential oil

Actions: aphrodisiac, astringent, bitter, relaxing nervine

Uses in pregnancy: Drops of jasmine oil can be used in massage rubs or added to a defuser for postnatal depression. As a uterine stimulant it also helps regulate contractions during labor, and its scent will help create a relaxing, loving atmosphere in the birthing room.

Kelp (*Fucus vesiculosis, Ascophyllum nodosum, Laminaria* spp., et.)

Various species of seaweed are sold commercially as "kelp" although herbalists usually regard *Fucus vesiculosis* as the main source. All are salty, tonic herbs, rich in iodine, trace metals, and other essential nutrients. The iodine content stimulates the thyroid and thus speeds up body metabolism; hence kelp's reputation as a slimming aid. Externally, bladderwrack oil can be used for rheumatic and arthritic problems.

Parts used: whole plant (thalli)

Actions: metabolic stimulant, nutritive, thyroid tonic, antirheumatic, anti-inflammatory

Uses in pregnancy: Kelp is a good mineral source for use in anemia; it can be helpful after the birth if there is general debility and weakness.

Caution: Bladderwrack can concentrate toxic waste metals such as cadmium and strontium which pollute our oceans, and should not be collected in contaminated areas.

Lady's mantle   (*Alchemilla xanthoclora*)

Lady's mantle is rich in tannins, so it is a good astringent, useful for diarrhea, sore throats, bleeding gums, and skin sores. It has a gynecological action and is used in parts of Europe as a menstrual regulator, especially for heavy periods, or in ointments for vaginal itching.

Parts used: aerial parts, leaves

Actions: astringent, menstrual regulator, digestive tonic, anti-inflammatory, wound herb

Uses in pregnancy: Lady's mantle will normalize and stimulate the menstrual cycle, so it can be helpful for infertility. In the final weeks of pregnancy, it can help to strengthen the womb for childbirth.

Caution: Avoid high doses during early pregnancy as it is a uterine stimulant.

Lavender   (*Lavandula angustifolia*)

The name "lavender" comes from the Latin *lavare*, meaning "to wash," and the herb has been used to scent baths and toiletries since Roman times. It is a very relaxing herb, ideal for nervous tension and insomnia.

Parts used: flowers, essential oil

Actions: analgesic, antibacterial, antidepressant, antispasmodic, carminative, bile stimulant, circulatory stimulant, relaxant, tonic for the nervous system

Uses in pregnancy: Diluted lavender oil makes a good massage for back pains, to help combat edema, or to ease birthing pains. The oil can also be diluted in warm water to make an antiseptic wash for perineal tears; add it to wheat germ oil as a massage during pregnancy to help avoid stretch marks. Drinking lavender tea is calming and relaxing for anxiety. The infusion can also be used as a wash for the perineum or in hot compresses to ease breast engorgement when nursing.

Lemon (*Citrus limonum*)

Lemons were considered an antidote for poisons by the Romans and are still used to combat infection. They are a rich source of many minerals and vitamins including B_1, B_2, B_3, C, and carotene (provitamin A).

Parts used: fruit, essential oil

Actions: antibacterial, anti-inflammatory, antihistamine, antirheumatic, antiscorbutic, antiseptic, antiviral, carminative, cleansing, cooling, diuretic, tonifying for heart and blood vessels

Uses in pregnancy: Lemons can improve the peripheral circulation and, as a venous tonic, may be helpful for hemorrhoids and varicose veins. The oil can also be used in massage rubs to combat edema.

Lemon balm (*Melissa officinalis*)

"Melissa" comes from the Greek word *mel*, meaning "honey," and the herb has a long association with bees and the healing power of their products. The sixteenth-century herbalist Paracelsus considered it an "elixir of youth."

Parts used: aerial parts, essential oil

Actions: antibacterial, antidepressant, antiviral, diaphoretic, digestive stimulant, peripheral vasodilator, relaxing restorative for nervous system, sedative

Uses in pregnancy: Lemon balm will ease all sorts of digestive upsets, including morning sickness. It is an ideal gentle sedative for emotional upsets but is also potent enough to help with postnatal depression.

Licorice *(Glycyrrhiza glabra)*

Licorice is one of our most widely researched and respected medicinal herbs; extracts are still widely used in orthodox drugs for digestive problems. The plant also has a hormonal effect, stimulating the adrenal cortex and encouraging production of such hormones as hydrocortisone.

Part used: root

Actions: antiarthritic, anti-inflammatory, antispasmodic, cooling, lowers cholesterol levels, expectorant, mild laxative, soothing for gastric mucosa, tonic stimulant for adrenal cortex, possibly anti-allergenic

Uses in pregnancy: Licorice is one of the safer laxative remedies for treating constipation.

Caution: Excessive licorice can cause fluid retention and increase blood pressure, so should be avoided by those suffering from hypertension or taking digoxin-based drugs.

Lime *(Tilia cordata)*

Lime flowers are used as a popular after-dinner tea (or tisane) in France taken to encourage relaxation and improve the digestion. They are also believed to combat the buildup of fatty plaques on blood vessels which can lead to arteriosclerosis.

Part used: flowers

Actions: antispasmodic, diaphoretic, diuretic, sedative, anticoagulant, immune stimulant, digestive remedy

Uses in pregnancy: Lime flowers can safely be used for high blood pressure and make a relaxing tea for anxiety and emotional upsets. Introduce the herb to babies as a dilute infusion by bottle; they'll like the taste and it will help later teething pains.

Marigold (*Calendula officinalis*)

Pot marigolds have been among the herbalist's favorites for centuries. In the twelfth century simply looking at the plant's golden color was supposed to lift the spirits and encourage cheerfulness.

Part used: flowers

Actions: astringent, antiseptic, antifungal, anti-inflammatory, antispasmodic, bitter, bile stimulant, diaphoretic, immune stimulant, menstrual regulator, wound herb

Uses in pregnancy: Marigold is a valuable gynecological herb for stimulating the menstrual cycle in infertility and can be used in an abdominal compress to ease birthing pains. Over-the-counter marigold creams, often sold as "calendula," are an ideal soothing and antiseptic remedy for vaginal thrush, perineal tears, or diaper rash; alternatively, you can use the infusion as a wash or bath. The herb is an essential standby in breast-feeding; use the cream for sore nipples or a compress to ease mastitis and engorgement. A homemade cold infused oil is a good alternative to over-the-counter ointments.

Marshmallow (*Althaea officinale*)

Marshmallow is a soothing, mucilaginous herb used to ease such ailments as bronchitis, irritating coughs, and cystitis; the root is especially soothing to the digestive system. Externally, it is used for various skin problems and has a soothing, softening effect on the skin.

Parts used: root, leaves, flowers

Actions: Root and leaves: demulcent, expectorant, diuretic, wound herb; *Flowers:* expectorant

Uses in pregnancy: A maceration of marshmallow root or tablets of the powdered herb are ideal for easing heartburn and indigestion.

Meadowsweet (*Filipendula ulmaria*)

Meadowsweet's best-known claim to fame is as the herb that gave us the name "aspirin." In the 1890s, the researchers at the German drug company Bayer named their new drug after the old botanical name for meadowsweet (*Spiraea ulmaria*) since both contained similar chemicals.

Parts used: whole plant collected when flowering

Actions: mild analgesic, antacid, anti-inflammatory, antirheumatic, antiseptic, astringent, diaphoretic, diuretic, soothing for the gastric membranes

Uses in pregnancy: Unlike aspirin, meadowsweet is extremely soothing and calming to the digestive tract, so it is ideal for gastritis, indigestion, and heartburn. It can also be useful to ease the discomfort of hiatal hernia. Just as a daily aspirin tablet is now often used to reduce the risk of preeclampsia, herbalists have long recommended a daily cup of meadowsweet infusion.

Caution: Meadowsweet is best avoided by those sensitive to salicylates and aspirin.

Melilot (*Melilotus officinale*)

Melilot smells of new-mown hay, due to the coumarins it contains, which account for much of its antithrombotic action. It is useful for easing the pain and eczema associated with varicose veins and can also be helpful for facial neuralgia or in eyebaths for conjunctivitis.

Parts used: aerial parts

Actions: anticoagulant, antithrombotic, antispasmodic, anti-inflammatory, diuretic, expectorant, sedative, styptic, mild analgesic

Uses in pregnancy: Melilot can be used internally and externally for varicose veins and hemorrhoids.

Caution: Do not take melilot if using anticoagulant drugs such as warfarin.

Milk thistle (*Silybum marianum*)

Milk thistle is a highly regarded protective remedy for the liver; it contains silymarin (which has been shown to prevent toxic chemicals from damaging liver tissue) and has been successfully used to treat cirrhosis and hepatitis.

Parts used: leaves, seeds

Actions: bitter tonic, protects the liver, stimulates bile flow, increases milk flow, antidepressant, antiviral

Uses in pregnancy: Drink an infusion of the leaves to stimulate milk flow when breast-feeding.

Motherwort (*Leonurus cardiaca*)

Motherwort is generally used as a heart tonic and sedative, although it takes its name from its traditional use in childbirth. Recent research also suggests it can help prevent thrombosis. It is popular for treating menopausal upsets and premenstrual syndrome.

Parts used: aerial parts

Actions: uterine stimulant, relaxant, cardiac tonic, carminative

Uses in pregnancy: Drink motherwort tea during labor to calm anxiety and stimulate the womb. The tea can also be used in the month before the baby is due to help prepare the womb for childbirth.

Caution: Avoid high doses during pregnancy, except in the final weeks or during labor, as it is a uterine stimulant.

Mugwort (*Artemisia vulgaris*)

Mugwort was reputedly planted alongside roads by the Romans who liked to put sprigs in their sandals to prevent their feet from aching on long journeys. In China, mugwort leaves are used as *moxa*; this means they are made into sticks of dried herb to be burned at the end of acupuncture needles (moxibustion) for "cold" conditions such as arthritis.

Parts used: aerial parts

Actions: stimulates the appetite, bitter, diaphoretic, diuretic, menstrual regulator, nervine, reduces cholesterol levels

Uses in pregnancy: Mugwort is used in traditional Chinese formulas to combat threatened miscarriage. It can relieve abdominal cramps and is useful during birthing to stimulate and regulate contractions.

Caution: Do not take in pregnancy (unless under professional guidance) or when breast-feeding.

Neroli (*Citrus aurantium*)

In the sixteenth century, an Italian princess (Anna-Marie de Nerola) reputedly discovered an oil extracted from orange blossoms that she used to scent her gloves. The oil took her name (neroli), and is now one of the most prized and highly priced aromatics. The typical cost is more than $500 a liter (rather expensive to lavish on gloves).

Part used: essential oil

Actions: antidepressant, sedative, tonic, antiseptic, antispasmodic

Uses in pregnancy: Drops of neroli oil can be added to massage rubs and bathwater for postnatal depression. The oil also makes a luxurious addition to wheat germ massage oil used to prevent stretch marks.

Nutmeg (*Myristica fragrans*)

Despite its familiarity as a kitchen seasoning, nutmeg is actually quite a potent hallucinogen and soporific with cases of delirium as a result of overconsumption reported as early as 1576. In low doses it is ideal for digestive problems such as nausea, abdominal bloating, indigestion, and colic.

Parts used: seed kernel (nutmeg), aril (mace), essential oil

Actions: carminative, digestive stimulant, antispasmodic, antiemetic, appetite stimulant, anti-inflammatory

Uses in pregnancy: Nutmeg oil is a traditional Eastern remedy used in abdominal massage to ease and encourage childbirth.

Caution: Large doses (5 grams or more in a single dose) can produce convulsions; avoid in pregnancy.

Oak (*Quercus* spp.)

Q. robur, the English or common oak, is helpful for many conditions involving bleeding or discharge including diarrhea, hemorrhage, minor injuries, weeping eczema, and vaginal discharges.

Q. alba, the North American white oak, was soon adopted for use in similar ways by the early settlers.

Part used: bark

Actions: astringent, antiseptic, anti-inflammatory, styptic

Uses in pregnancy: Oak decoctions can be used as a mouthwash for soft, bleeding gums or as an external lotion for varicose veins and hemorrhoids. Drinking the mix as a tea is also helpful.

Oats (*Avena sativa*)

Oats are one of the world's most important cereal crops, used as a staple food in northern Europe for centuries. They are sweet, nutritious, and warming and are rich in iron, zinc, and manganese, and so are a good source of many vital minerals.

Parts used: seeds and grain extracts, whole plant

Actions: antidepressant, restorative nerve tonic, diaphoretic, nutritive; the bran is antithrombotic and lowers cholesterol levels.

Uses in pregnancy: Eat hot oatmeal as a gentle restorative and stimulant for the nervous system and to combat postnatal depression. Alternatively, take oat straw tincture or juice of fresh oats, pressed when still green.

Parsley (*Petroselinum crispum*)

Although more familiar as a garnish, parsley is also a valuable medicinal herb and is a good source of vitamins and minerals, a useful addition to the diet for anemia. It is often employed as a diuretic for premenstrual fluid retention and is a cleansing remedy for rheumatism. Chewing fresh parsley reputedly reduces the lingering smell of garlic.

Parts used: leaves, roots, seeds

Actions: antispasmodic, antirheumatic, diuretic, carminative, expectorant, tonic, antimicrobial, nutrient

Uses in pregnancy: Parsley is a good source of minerals; eat the fresh leaves to help combat cramps and anemia. An occasional cup of tea can also be used to reduce fluid retention.

Caution: Avoid the seeds or high doses of the leaves in pregnancy.

Passion flower (*Passiflora incarnata*)

Passion flower takes its name from the religious symbolism of its flowers rather than any therapeutic effects. It was traditionally used by Native Americans as a tonic and was initially utilized in Europe as a remedy for epilepsy and later for insomnia.

Parts used: aerial parts

Actions: mild analgesic, antispasmodic, hypnotic, mild sedative, vasodilator

Uses in pregnancy: As a gentle sedative, passion flower will ease anxiety and stress as well as insomnia. It will also reduce blood pressure and steady an irregular heartbeat.

Patchouli (*Pogostemon cablin*)

Originating from Malaysia where it was used as a stimulant and insecticide, patchouli oil is thick and dark brown, often with a greenish tinge. Its scent is strong and lingering, and it is not universally liked, so experiment carefully before using large amounts.

Part used: essential oil

Actions: antidepressant, anti-inflammatory, astringent, antiseptic, cell regenerator

Uses in pregnancy: Drops of patchouli can be added to massage rubs for postnatal depression or, if you like the smell, added to a defuser. It is also popular in massage treatments for edema and fluid retention.

Peppermint *(Mentha X piperita)*

Peppermint is believed to be a cross between spearmint (*M. spicata*) and water mint (*M. aquatica*); it has a high menthol content, hence the characteristic smell. Spearmint is most often grown in gardens and makes an adequate substitute, especially during pregnancy.

Parts used: leaves

Actions: analgesic, antiemetic, antispasmodic, carminative, bile stimulant, digestive tonic, peripheral vasodilator, diaphoretic (but also cooling internally)

Uses in pregnancy: Although peppermint is popular to ease morning sickness, the menthol can be an irritant and a uterine stimulant, so avoid large or regular doses and do not take the oil. A few drops of peppermint emulsion are ideal for disguising the flavor of less pleasant herbs.

Caution: Peppermint in any form should not be given to babies or toddlers; it can irritate the stomach lining, and misuse may lead to ulceration. The herb can also cause an allergic reaction in sensitive individuals.

Pilewort *(Ranunculus ficaria)*

Pilewort is generally regarded as a classic example of the medieval Doctrine of Signatures: the plant's roots are full of tiny nodules that resemble bunches of grapes, or more prosaically, piles, so the herb was recommended as a remedy for hemorrhoids and given its common name. It contains protoanemonin, which is an irritant, but is destroyed by drying, so fresh pilewort should be avoided.

Parts used: whole plant

Actions: astringent, demulcent

Uses in pregnancy: Externally, creams and washes will soothe the irritation and soreness of hemorrhoids; pilewort taken internally will have a similar effect.

Plantain *(Plantago major)*

Common plantain, a familiar garden weed, has long been regarded as an important healing herb. The fresh leaves will ease insect bites, while internally it can be used for gastric upsets, irritable bowel syndrome, heavy menstrual periods, and cystitis.

Part used: leaves

Actions: antibacterial, antihistamine, antiallergenic, astringent, blood tonic, demulcent, diuretic, expectorant, styptic

Uses in pregnancy: Drink the tea to ease hemorrhoids and use it externally as a wash or compress for both hemorrhoids and perineal tears.

Raspberry *(Rubus idaeus)*

Raspberry leaf is best known for its tonifying effect on the uterus and its use as a preparative for childbirth. It will also ease menstrual pains, is an effective gargle for sore throats, and may be taken for diarrhea.

Parts used: leaves, fruit

Actions: astringent, *partus praeparator*, stimulant, digestive remedy, tonic, diuretic, laxative

Uses in pregnancy: Drink the infusion during the last six weeks of pregnancy to prepare the womb for childbirth. The same mix will also ease the discomfort and contractions associated with afterpains.

Caution: Avoid high doses of the leaves during the first six months of pregnancy.

Red clover (*Trifolium pratense*)

Red clover is used by herbalists mainly as a cleansing remedy for skin problems such as psoriasis and eczema. It is a useful expectorant and diuretic, helpful for dry coughs and gout, while the fresh flowers can relieve insect bites and stings.

Part used: flowers

Actions: cleansing, antispasmodic, diuretic, possible estrogenic activity

Uses in pregnancy: Red clover is an excellent breast remedy and was used in the 1930s for breast cancer. Internally, or as a compress, it can ease mastitis, while the tea is a good tonic for the female reproductive system if infertility is a problem.

Rose (*Rosa* spp.)

The rose is probably one of the West's most neglected medicinal herbs, although until the 1930s it was regularly prescribed for sore throats and diarrhea. Rose hips are still valued as an important source of vitamin C, and rose oil is used for skin and emotional problems. Various varieties of rose are used in Chinese medicine as tonics and for liver and menstrual disorders.

Parts used: petals, rose hips, essential oil, leaves

Actions: antidepressant, antispasmodic, aphrodisiac, astringent, sedative, digestive stimulant, bile stimulant, cleansing, expectorant, antibacterial, antiviral, antiseptic

Uses in pregnancy: Rose oil is a powerful remedy for the emotions and nervous system; in massage or baths it will help ease postnatal depression. It is also good for the skin; add it to remedies for sore nipples. The infused petals and leaves are astringent to ease such conditions as varicose veins, while rose hips are a good source of vitamin C to improve iron absorption in anemia.

Rose geranium (*Pelargonium graveolens*)

Rose geranium oil was originally produced at Grasse in France, but as labor costs increased, production migrated first to Algeria and later to the island of Réunion in the Indian Ocean. This island was then known as Île Bourbon, so the oil became known as "Bourbon oil." It is particularly rich in citronellol which makes it a useful insect repellent.

Part used: essential oil

Actions: antidepressant, antiseptic, astringent, diuretic, styptic, stimulates the adrenal cortex

Uses in pregnancy: Drops of rose geranium oil can be added to wheat germ oil to make a pleasant rub to use throughout pregnancy to prevent stretch marks. It is also useful in massages for swollen ankles and fluid retention or, well diluted, in compresses to ease breast swelling in mastitis and engorgement.

Rosemary (*Rosmarinus officinalis*)

Rosemary is traditionally associated with remembrance; sprigs were exchanged by lovers or scattered on coffins, and it does have a stimulating effect on the nervous system and memory.

Parts used: leaves, essential oil

Actions: Leaves: antiseptic, antidepressive, antispasmodic, astringent, cardiac tonic, carminative, bile stimulant, circulatory stimulant, diaphoretic, digestive remedy, diuretic, nervine, restorative tonic for nervous system; *Essential oil* (topically): analgesic, antirheumatic, rubefacient

Uses in pregnancy: Rosemary tea is a stimulating tonic for tiredness and debility following childbirth, while the essential oil can be used in massage rubs or baths to ease muscular pains and backache or can be sniffed to combat feelings of faintness.

Caution: Rosemary is a uterine stimulant in high doses. Do not take internally during pregnancy, although it is safe in culinary use.

Sage (*Salvia officinalis*)

Sage is traditionally associated with longevity and, like many folk traditions, this is yet another that modern research is verifying: the oil is a powerful antioxidant that combats the aging of the body's cells. The plant is also rich in estrogen and thus has a direct effect on the female reproductive system.

Parts used: leaves, essential oil

Actions: Leaves: antispasmodic, antiseptic, astringent, carminative, healing to mucosa, bile stimulant, lowers blood sugar levels, peripheral vasodilator, suppresses perspiration, reduces salivation and lactation, uterine stimulant, systemically antibiotic; *Essential oil:* antiseptic, antispasmodic, astringent, hypertensive, stimulant, emmenagogue, antioxidant

Uses in pregnancy: Sage oil is a traditional stimulant in childbirth and can be used in abdominal massage rubs during labor. Its hormonal action makes it ideal for relieving night sweats during menopause and for drying up milk in lactating mothers on weaning.

Sandalwood (*Santalum alba*)

Sandalwood is important in Ayurvedic medicine as a cooling herb that stimulates the mind and improves digestive energy. In aromatherapy the oil is regarded as relaxing and antidepressant; it is used for urinary problems, nervous disorders, and chest complaints and can be added to bathwater to encourage restful sleep.

Parts used: wood, essential oil

Actions: antiseptic, antibacterial, urinary antiseptic, carminative, relaxing, diuretic, antispasmodic

Uses in pregnancy: Sandalwood oil is helpful in postnatal depression. Use it in massage rubs, relaxing baths, or in a diffuser to scent the room.

Saw palmetto *(Serenoa repens)*

Saw palmetto berries originate in the southeastern United States and were traditionally highly valued for their tonic effect and used as a strengthening remedy in debility. Modern research has shown that the herb can combat prostate enlargement, but it is helpful for the female reproductive system as well.

Part used: berries

Actions: tonic, diuretic, sedative, urinary antiseptic, endocrine stimulant, hormonal action

Uses in pregnancy: Saw palmetto is a good male tonic for infertility, while its hormonal action also stimulates the mammary glands to increase milk production in nursing mothers.

Shepherd's purse *(Capsella bursa-pastoris)*

Shepherd's purse—also known as mother's hearts—is a persistent garden weed, but it has long been used in both Western and Chinese herbal traditions to stop hemorrhage. As an astringent and urinary antiseptic it is ideal for severe cystitis and is also used to normalize heavy menstrual flow.

Parts used: leaves, aerial parts

Actions: astringent, uterine relaxant, styptic, urinary antiseptic, circulatory stimulant, hypotensive

Uses in pregnancy: The infusion is helpful in labor to stimulate the womb and encourage regular contractions.

Caution: Avoid high doses in pregnancy, except during labor.

Sesame (*Sesamum indicum*)

The pungent, nutty flavor of sesame oil is well known from Chinese, Middle Eastern, and Indian cookery. Ground seeds, known as tahini, are an important flavoring in many traditions, and the seeds themselves are a good source of calcium.

Parts used: seeds, seed oil

Actions: antioxidant, demulcent, laxative, nutritive

Uses in pregnancy: As a good calcium source, eating plenty of sesame seeds can help combat cramps.

Siberian ginseng (*Eleutherococcus senticosus*)

Siberian ginseng is a comparative newcomer to the West, rediscovered in the 1930s in Russia and then extensively used by Soviet athletes to increase stamina and enhance performance. It has been extensively researched and is known to stimulate the immune and circulatory systems and also help regulate blood pressure.

Part used: root

Actions: adrenal stimulant, antiviral, adaptagen, aphrodisiac, combats the actions of stress, immune stimulant, lowers blood sugar levels, peripheral vasodilator, tonic

Uses in pregnancy: Siberian ginseng is ideal for helping the body cope with stress and combat fatigue. It can be taken at any time and is a safer tonic for regular use in pregnancy than Korean ginseng.

Skullcap (*Scutellaria lateriflora*)

Virginian skullcap was used by the Cherokee for encouraging menstruation, to treat diarrhea, and for breast pains. Today it is mainly considered as a sedative and nervine by Western herbalists, but it can also be used to reduce fevers, calm the fetus, and stimulate digestion.

Parts used: aerial parts

Actions: antibacterial, antispasmodic, cooling, digestive stimulant, hypotensive, lowers cholesterol levels, relaxing and restorative nervine, styptic

Uses in pregnancy: Skullcap tea will combat anxiety and nervous tension and also help with insomnia and emotional upsets. It can be useful for stress-related blood pressure problems and is a good mineral source for anemia.

Slippery elm (*Ulmus rubra*)

The bark of the slippery or red elm was one of the most widely used of Native American medicines. The Ozark Indians took it for colds and bowel complaints, while the Missouri Valley tribes used a decoction as a laxative. The bark is highly mucilaginous and provides a protective coating for the stomach, so it will soothe the mucous membranes in gastritis and ulceration.

Part used: bark

Actions: antitussive, cleansing, demulcent, expectorant, healing, nutrient; topically as an emollient

Uses in pregnancy: Slippery elm can help ease digestive upsets contributing to morning sickness and is ideal for heartburn. It is also a useful dietary supplement in debility and convalescence.

Spearmint (*Mentha spicata*)

The familiar garden mint that so often accompanies roast lamb is usually a variety of spearmint. It is much gentler than peppermint and is mainly used for minor problems, such as gas and indigestion, and also for children's fevers and stomach upsets.

Parts used: leaves, oil

Actions: antispasmodic, carminative, diaphoretic, stimulant

Uses in pregnancy: Drink an infusion for indigestion and heartburn and try it as an alternative to peppermint for morning sickness.

Squaw vine (*Mitchella repens*)

Although Native Americans used squaw vine, also known as partridge berry, for insomnia and as a diuretic, the main use was to ease labor pains and in the weeks before the birth to help prepare the womb.

Parts used: whole plant

Actions: astringent, diuretic, parturient, uterine tonic, stimulant

Uses in pregnancy: Squaw vine combines well with raspberry leaf as a regular infusion in the weeks before the birth. It can also be taken throughout labor and can help after the birth to speed contraction of the uterus. Externally, the infusion can be used as a wash for sore nipples during breast-feeding.

St. John's wort (*Hypericum perforatum*)

St. John's wort has hit the headlines in recent years as a powerful antidepressant and an immune stimulant used in AIDS treatment. Traditionally it was used as a wound herb and is a useful home remedy for cuts, burns, and scrapes.

Parts used: flowering tops collected in midsummer, leaves collected before or after flowering

Actions: astringent, analgesic, anti-inflammatory, antidepressant, sedative, restorative tonic for the nervous system

Uses in pregnancy: Externally, St. John's wort is useful after the birth to heal perineal tears and discomfort. Internally, the infusion will help insomnia and nervous tension while as an antidepressant it is ideal for postnatal blues. The infused oil is also anti-inflammatory, so it makes a good base for massage rubs for muscular aches and back pain; drinking the tea will help too.

Caution: Prolonged use may increase photosensitivity of the skin in rare cases. Prolonged depression generally requires professional help; do not depend on self-help remedies.

Stinging nettle (*Urtica dioica*)

Stinging nettles were once used in a rather bizarre treatment known as urtication, which involved beating paralyzed limbs with stinging nettles in an attempt to stimulate sensations. Thanks to its ability to "rob the soil" and concentrate minerals and vitamins in its leaves, nettle is a good supplement for iron-deficiency anemia.

Parts used: aerial parts, root

Actions: antiseptic, antirheumatic, astringent, blood tonic, diuretic, expectorant, galactagogue, hypotensive, lowers blood sugar levels, important source of minerals, clears uric acid

Uses in pregnancy: As well as providing important minerals and vitamins for anemia and cramps, stinging nettles are a good general tonic that can be useful to combat infertility associated with debility and weakness. The herb stimulates milk flow, so nettle tea is a good drink for nursing mothers as well.

Tea tree (*Melaleuca alternifolia*)

Extracts from the Australian tea tree were originally used by the Aborigines as a wound remedy. The plant was first studied in Europe in the 1920s when French researchers found that the oil, collected by steam distillation, was a more effective antiseptic than phenol, and identified its impressive antibiotic properties.

Part used: essential oil

Actions: antibacterial, antifungal, antiseptic, antiviral, diaphoretic, expectorant

Uses in pregnancy: Tea tree oil is ideal externally for any sorts of skin sores and infections—from cuts and scrapes to thrush. Dilute the oil in water and use as a wash to counter bladder infections or for diaper rash.

Uva-ursi (*Arctostaphylos uva-ursi*)

Uva-ursi or bearberry is a small, evergreen shrub from northern Europe widely used for treating cystitis and similar complaints. It contains the chemical arbutin, which is very antiseptic for the entire urinary tract.

Part used: leaves

Actions: antibacterial, astringent, urinary antiseptic

Uses in pregnancy: The infusion is ideal for cystitis and similar problems. Although often recommended for fluid retention, uva-ursi is only mildly diuretic so it is not the remedy of choice.

Vervain (*Verbena officinalis*)

Vervain is mainly used as a nervine and liver tonic; it is bitter and stimulating for the digestion and makes an ideal tonic in convalescence and debility. Externally, it can ease the pain of neuralgia.

Parts used: aerial parts

Actions: relaxant tonic, stimulates milk production, diaphoretic, nervine, sedative, antispasmodic, hepatic restorative, laxative, uterine stimulant, bile stimulant

Uses in pregnancy: As a milk stimulant, vervain tea is ideal in breast-feeding and can also be taken in labor to regulate and ease contractions. As an antidepressant, it can also be helpful for postnatal problems.

Caution: Avoid in pregnancy, although it can be taken in labor.

Watercress (*Nasturtium officinale*)

Familiar in salads and soups, watercress is also a medicinal plant that will stimulate the digestion, liver function, and kidney metabolism and act as a valuable cleansing remedy for skin problems. Combined with nettle juice it makes a good "spring cleaning" potion used as a restorative after the winter.

Part used: leaves

Actions: antiscorbutic, blood enricher, reduces blood sugar levels, diuretic, expectorant

Uses in pregnancy: Eating plenty of watercress is a simple way to prevent anemia; juice the fresh herb in a food processor and take 2 teaspoons daily. It is also a diuretic, so it can be helpful for easing fluid retention and for lowering high blood pressure.

White willow (*Salix alba*)

The *Salix* genus gives its name to "salicylates," the group of anti-inflammatory and analgesic compounds found in aspirin and present in significant amounts in the bark and leaves of the white willow. The plant, like aspirin, is used for relieving pain, reducing fevers, and easing rheumatism, gout, arthritis, feverish chills, and headaches.

Part used: bark

Actions: antirheumatic, anti-inflammatory, antipyretic, antihidrotic, analgesic, antiseptic, astringent, bitter digestive tonic

Uses in pregnancy: Like aspirin and meadowsweet, white willow can be taken as a daily tea if there is any risk of preeclampsia; it helps to combat clotting and thickening of the placental blood supply.

Caution: Avoid if allergic to salicylates.

Wild yam (*Dioscorea villosa*)

Rich in steroidal saponins, wild yam's main claim to fame is as the original source of the oral contraceptive pill. It is largely used for colic and rheumatism but can also be taken for menstrual pain, cramps, asthma, gastritis, and gallbladder problems.

Parts used: root, rhizome

Actions: relaxant for smooth muscle, antispasmodic, stimulates bile flow, anti-inflammatory, mild diaphoretic

Uses in pregnancy: The decoction or tincture can be used in childbirth to stimulate contractions and is also helpful later to relieve afterpains and the discomfort of involution.

Cautions: May cause nausea in high doses.

Winter cherry/ Ashwagandha (*Withania somnifera*)

Known as *ashwagandha* in Hindi, withania or winter cherry is an important Ayurvedic tonic believed to increase vitality and clear the mind. It is mainly used in the West as a tonic to combat debility resulting from overwork and chronic stress, although in India it is also used as a tonic in pregnancy.

Part used: root

Actions: tonic, sedative, combats stress

Uses in pregnancy: Winter cherry is a useful tonic for both partners; it can be especially effective where male fertility is a problem.

Witch hazel (*Hamamelis virginiana*)

Witch hazel was popular with many Native American tribes: the Menomee Indians in Wisconsin rubbed decoctions on their legs to keep the muscles supple, while the Potawatomis preferred the twigs in steam baths. The bark is steam-distilled to produce the familiar clear "distilled witch hazel" available from any pharmacy.

Part used: bark

Actions: astringent, anti-inflammatory, styptic

Uses in pregnancy: Distilled witch hazel is astringent and healing for perineal soreness, hemorrhoids, and varicose veins. The tincture is stronger and can be used diluted with water or make an infusion of the leaves and use as a wash.

Wood betony (*Stachys officinalis*)

Although held in high regard by the Anglo-Saxons, who had some twenty-nine medicinal uses for the plant, wood betony has now fallen from fashion. It is an excellent remedy for headaches and nervous upsets, useful for liver and respiratory disorders, and makes a pleasant tea for everyday drinking.

Parts used: aerial parts

Actions: sedative, bitter digestive remedy, nervine, circulatory tonic particularly for cerebral circulation, astringent

Uses in pregnancy: Wood betony is a restorative and supportive tea to drink during labor; it helps to regulate contractions as well as to calm anxieties and tension.

Caution: Avoid in pregnancy except during labor.

Yellow dock (*Rumex crispus*)

Yellow dock is a cleansing herb suitable for chronic skin problems and arthritic complaints. It is also a laxative and stimulates bowel flow but is gentler than strong purgatives such as rhubarb root or senna.

Part used: root

Actions: laxative, bile stimulant, cleansing

Uses in pregnancy: Yellow dock is rich in iron and makes a helpful supplement for anemia. It is also one of the gentler laxatives to use for constipation in pregnancy; however, it should be used in moderation.

11
How to Prepare Herbal Remedies

Making your own herbal remedies is no more difficult than blending sauces or cooking vegetables. Basic kitchen equipment is all that is needed, although if remedies are to be kept for any length of time, it is important to use sterile bottles and jars for storage. This section details simple methods for making the sorts of remedies that may be of use during pregnancy and childbirth. More complex products, such as creams, ointments, and capsules, are available ready-made from health food stores and pharmacies.

Infusions

An infusion is simply a tea made by steeping the herb in freshly boiled water for ten minutes; it is an ideal method for most leafy herbs and flowers. Typically use 1 to 2 teaspoons of herb to a cup of water (1 cup = 8 fluid ounces). Put the herb into a ceramic or glass teapot, jar, or cup (with lid) and bring the water just up to a boil (otherwise, many aromatic plant constituents will be lost in the excessive steam); pour the water over the herbs, cover, and let steep for ten minutes. After infusing, strain through a sieve. Drink a cup three times a day; sweeten with a little honey, if desired.

If using fresh herbs, you need three times as much herb per cup of water to allow for the additional weight of water in the fresh plant material.

Although the infusion can be reheated before each dose, it is best to make only enough infusion for one dose or one day's dosages at a time. If necessary, surplus can be stored in the refrigerator for up to forty-eight hours.

Decoctions

A decoction is also a tea but is made by simmering the plant material for fifteen to twenty minutes; it is ideal for tougher components such as barks, roots, and berries, where it can be more difficult to extract the active ingredients. Use 1 to 2 teaspoons of herb to 1½ cups of cold water, which should then be brought to a boil in a stainless steel, glass, ceramic, or enamel saucepan (not aluminum) and allowed to simmer until the volume has been reduced by about a third.

The mixture is then strained through a sieve and taken in cup doses during the day. Decoctions can be reduced after straining to between 1 to 2 tablespoons with further gentle heating. Then this concentrated mix can be used in drop dosages, either alone or in water. This can be a good way to administer decoctions to children, who are often reluctant to drink whole cups of herbal brews.

Combined Infusions and Decoctions

When using a number of herbs in a tea it is often necessary to use some as infusions and some as decoctions; for example, a tea of ginger root with elder flowers and yarrow for a cold. In these cases it is best to measure out the required 1½ cups of water (or 4½ cups if making enough for the day) and use this to simmer the required amount of roots (usually ½ to 1 teaspoon per dose). Once the volume has reduced by about a third, pour the still simmering mixture over the dried leaves and flowers, in a teapot or cup, cover, and infuse for a further ten to fifteen minutes. Strain and drink.

Infused Oils

Infused oils can be used as a base for massage and abdominal rubs. There are two techniques: hot infusion or cold infusion.

Hot infused oils: These are made by heating 2 cups of dried herb in 1 pint of sunflower (or similar) oil in a double boiler over water for about three hours. Remember to refill the lower saucepan with hot water from time to time to prevent it from boiling dry. After about three hours the oil will take on a greenish color; it can then be strained and squeezed through a muslin bag and stored in clean glass bottles, away from direct sunlight. This method is suitable for making infused comfrey or rosemary oil.

Cold infused oils: Because the oil is not heated in this method, you can use good-quality seed oils that are rich in essential fatty acids (EFAs), which have significant therapeutic properties. Oils high in EFA include walnut, safflower, and pumpkin oils. The cold infused oil is made by simply filling a large screw-top jar (such as a clean coffee jar) with the dried or fresh herb and then completely covering it with oil. The jar should be left on a sunny windowsill for at least three weeks; the mixture can then be strained through a muslin bag. The cold infused method is suitable for St. John's wort, marigold, or chamomile flowers.

Massage Oils

The massage oils used in aromatherapy are very easy to make at home by adding a few drops of essential oil to some sort of oil base. Suitable bases include sweet almond oil, wheat germ oil, avocado oil, or any of the infused herb oils made from walnut or sunflower oil described above.

In general, do not use more than 10 percent essential oil (10 drops of essential oil in a teaspoon of carrier oil), as many essential oils can irritate sensitive skin. Always buy good-quality organically grown essential oils; many cheaper ones are chemically adulterated or contain pollutants.

Compresses

Compresses are often used to ease muscle cramps and discomfort. They are basically cloth pads soaked in herbal extracts and applied hot to painful limbs, swellings, or strains. Use a clean piece of cotton, cotton wool, linen, or surgical gauze soaked in a hot, strained infusion, decoction, or tincture (diluted with hot water) and apply to the affected area. When the compress cools repeat using fresh, hot mixture.

Occasionally a cold compress may be used, as with some perineal tears when a cool pad soaked in St. John's wort infusion can be helpful.

Poultices

Poultices have a very similar action to compresses but involve directly applying the whole herb to an affected area rather than using a liquid extract. Generally hot poultices are applied to swellings and sprains or to draw pus or splinters.

In pregnancy, cabbage leaf or plantain poultices are an effective remedy for mastitis. Simply bruise fresh herbs or mix in a food processor for a few seconds; then spread the mixture onto gauze and apply to the breast. Mix dried herbs or powders with hot water to make a paste; then squeeze out any surplus liquid and spread the residue on gauze or apply directly to the area affected.

Tinctures

Tinctures contain alcohol, which some women wish to avoid totally during pregnancy. They are, however, a convenient way of taking herbs; adding a little very hot water to each dose and then leaving it to cool will evaporate off the bulk of the alcohol present.

Tinctures are made by soaking the dried or fresh plant material in a mixture of alcohol and water for two weeks and then straining the mix through a wine press or jelly bag. Commercially produced tinctures are usually made from ethyl alcohol, which can be difficult to obtain for general use. *Caution:* Never use industrial alcohol (methyl alcohol) or rubbing alcohol (isopropyl alcohol); they are toxic and must be avoided. Glycerol can be used instead of alcohol. It is much less expensive, but the resulting tinctures are slightly slimy to the taste. For home use, probably the safest and most accessible source of alcohol is in the liquor cabinet—spirits and wines.

Most tinctures are made from a mixture containing 25 percent alcohol in water (for example, 1 cup of pure alcohol with 3 cups of water). This is slightly weaker in strength than most proof spirits, so a suitable mixture can easily be made by diluting over-the-counter drinks. Vodka is generally considered the most suitable as it has few other flavorings or herbal ingredients. For a 37.5 percent alcohol mixture, simply use half as much water; for every 2 cups of vodka, add 1 cup of water; this makes a 25 percent alcohol/water mixture that can then be used for tincture making.

Standard tinctures are usually made in the weight-to-volume proportion 1/5 (for example, 1 pound of herb to 5 pints of liquid). For domestic use, mixing 2 cups of dried herb with 2½ pints of liquid is usually a sufficient quantity to make at any one time. If using fresh herb, use three times as much herb to account for the water content of the herb (for example, 6 cups of fresh herb to 2½ pints of liquid).

To make the tincture, simply put the required quantity of herb into a large jar (such as a well-washed large glass screw-top coffee jar). Then cover with the alcohol/water mixture and store in a cool place for two weeks, shaking the bottle occasionally. Strain the mixture through a wine press or jelly bag and store the resulting liquid in clean, dark glass containers. The tincture will generally keep for up to two years without deterioration. In general, tinctures are taken in 1 teaspoon doses up to three times a day.

Some herbs—mainly roots, barks, or those that contain a lot of resins or essential oils—need to be extracted in 45 to 60 percent alcohol mixtures (difficult to obtain for home use), so these are best bought over the counter.

Buying and Storing Herbs

Always buy herbs in small quantities (½ to 1 pound at a time) to ensure freshness; if possible, examine the herbs before buying to check on quality. Choose herbs that have a good color and aroma and are not faded; they should not have a musty smell. Avoid shops that display herbs in clear glass jars on sunny shelves—the quality will probably be poor. Inadequate storage can lead to rapid deterioration with mouse droppings, mold, and insects among unwanted pollutants.

Ideally, buy organic herbs or those labeled "wild crafted," which means they have been collected in the wild rather than grown as a commercial—and often heavily sprayed—cash crop. Poor harvesting can lead to many unwanted additions; dried grass, for example, is often found with herbs such as eyebright, which have been gathered from meadow areas. With practice one can soon recognize the characteristics of many dried herbs, so it becomes easier to check on the accuracy of labels. Agrimony, for example, has characteristic burrs (the seed heads), and many herbs can be identified from their aroma.

Herb Suppliers

Bay Laurel Farm
West Garzas Road
Camel Valley, CA 93924
(408) 659-2913

Frontier Cooperative Herbs
Box 299
Norway, IA 52318
1-800-669-3275

Herb Products Co.
11012 Magnolia Boulevard
North Hollywood, CA 91601
(818) 984-3141

Jean's Greens
119 Sulphur Springs Road
Newport, NY 13416
1-888-845-TEAS

Kiehls Pharmacy
109 Third Avenue
New York, NY 10009

May Way Trading
Chinese Herb Company
1338 Cypress Street
Oakland, CA 94607
(510) 208-3113

Sage Mountain Herbs
P.O. Box 420
East Barre, VT 05649
(802) 479-9825

Glossary

Adaptagen
A substance that helps the body to adapt to a new strain or stress by stimulating the body's defense mechanisms

Analgesic
Relieves pain

Anesthetic
Causes local or general loss of sensation

Anodyne
Allays pain

Antibacterial
Destroys or inhibits the growth of bacteria

Antibiotic
Destroys or inhibits the growth of microorganisms such as bacteria and fungi

Antifungal
Destroys or inhibits the growth of fungi

Anti-inflammatory
Reduces inflammation

Antimicrobial
Destroys or inhibits the growth of microorganisms such as bacteria and fungi

Antirheumatic
Relieves the symptoms of rheumatism

Antiseptic
Controls or prevents infection

Antispasmodic
Reduces muscle spasm and tension

Aphrodisiac
Promotes sexual excitement

Areola
The dark area around the nipple

Aril
Fleshy or hairy outgrowth of certain seeds

Astringent
Used to describe an herb that will precipitate proteins from the surface of cells or membranes causing tissues to contract and tighten; forms a protective coating and stops bleeding and discharges

Bach Flower Remedies
Extracts of flowers collected as dew and preserved in brandy, discovered by Dr. Edward Bach in the 1930s and widely used to treat emotional upsets and disturbances

Bitter
Stimulates secretion of digestive juices

Blood sugar
Levels of glucose in the blood

Bulk laxative
Increases the volume of feces, producing larger, softer stools

Carminative
Expels gas from the stomach and intestines to relieve flatulence, digestive colic, and gastric discomfort

***Chong* channel**
Also known as the "penetrating channel," the *Chong Mai* originates in the uterus and links all the main acupuncture meridians of the body

Circulatory stimulant
Increases blood flow

Cleansing herb
An herb that improves the excretion of waste products from the body

Colostrum
The rich, first breast milk full of important antibodies

Cooling
Used to describe herbs that are often bitter or relaxing and will help to reduce internal heat and hyperactivity

Demulcent
Softens and soothes damaged or inflamed surfaces, such as the gastric mucous membranes

Diaphoretic
Increases sweating

Diuretic
Encourages urine flow

Doctrine of Signatures
A medieval theory which argued that plants contained clues to their medicinal properties in their appearance; similar beliefs are found in most cultures worldwide

Emetic
Causes vomiting

Emmenagogue
Uterine stimulant that will encourage menstrual flow; excess may lead to miscarriage in pregnancy

Emollient
Softens and soothes the skin

Episiotomy
A routine surgical procedure in childbirth that involves cutting the perineum to avoid tears

Essential oil
Volatile chemicals extracted from plants by such techniques as steam distillation; highly active and aromatic

Febrifuge
Reduces fever

Fontanelle
Opening in the skull of the fetus or young baby due to incomplete ossification of the cranial bones and resulting in incomplete closure of the sutures; also known as the "soft spot"

Galactagogue
Increases production of breast milk

Hormone
A chemical substance produced in the body that can affect the way tissues behave; hormones can control sexual function as well as emotional and physical activity

Hyperacidity
Excessive digestive acid, causing a burning sensation

Hyperglycemic
Increases blood sugar levels

Hypertensive
Raises blood pressure

Hypoglycemic
Reduces blood sugar levels

Hypotensive
Lowers blood pressure

Hypotonic inertia
Stage in a protracted labor when the dilation of the cervix slows and contractions are weak and protracted

Involution
Contraction of the uterus after the birth, generally accompanied by cramping pains

Laxative
Encourages bowel motions

Mucilage
Complex sugar molecules found in plants that are soft and slippery and provide protection for the mucous membranes and inflamed surfaces

Neonate
A new baby, generally one younger than four weeks old

Nervine
Herb that affects the nervous system and that may be stimulating or sedating

Oxytocin
Hormone secreted by the pituitary gland that stimulates uterine contractions and milk ejection from lactating mammary glands

Partum praeparator
A substance which will help prepare the womb for childbirth

Perineum
The area between the anus and the vagina

Peripheral circulation
Blood supply to the limbs, skin, and muscles (including heart muscles)

Peristalsis
The waves of involuntary contractions in the digestive tract that move food and waste products through the system

Phlegm
Catarrhal-like secretion or sputum

Photosensitivity
Sensitivity to light

Pituitary gland
A major gland in the endocrine system controlling production of many vital hormones; located at the base of the skull

Postpartum
The period immediately following the birth

Progesterone
Steroid hormone produced in the ovary, placenta, and adrenal cortex that helps maintain the womb lining through pregnancy and prevents further release of eggs

Prolactin
Hormone produced by the pituitary gland that stimulates milk production

Pyrrolizidine alkaloids
Chemicals found in a number of plants (including comfrey and borage) which, in excess, can be associated with liver damage, although many regard the research evidence for this as inconclusive

Qi (ch'i)
The body's vital energy as defined in Chinese medicine

Relaxant
Relaxes tense and overactive nerves and tissues

Ren channel
Also known as the "conception vessel," the *Ren Mai* is an acupuncture meridian that arises in the uterus and is closely associated with the *yin* meridians in the body

Rubefacient
A substance that stimulates blood flow to the skin, causing local reddening

Sedative
Reduces anxiety and tension

Stimulant
Increases activity

Stria (pl. striae)
A faint ridge or streak; striation

Syntometrine
An ergometrine maleate, used routinely in the third stage of labor or after delivery to prevent postpartum hemorrhage

Styptic
Stops external bleeding

Systemic
Affecting the whole body

Tincture
Liquid herbal extract made by soaking plant material in a mixture of alcohol and water

Tonic
Restoring, nourishing, and supporting for the entire body

Tonify
Strengthening and restoring for the system

Topical
Local administration of an herbal remedy

Warming
A remedy that increases body temperature and encourages digestive function and circulation; warming herbs are often spicy and pungent to taste

Yang
Aspect of being equated with male energy: dry, hot, light, ascending

Yin
Aspect of being equated with female energy: damp, cold, dark, descending

References

Balaskas, J. 1998. *New Natural Pregnancy: Practical Well-Being from Conception to Birth*. London: Gaia Books.

Betz, J. M. et al. 1994. "Determination of pyrrolizidine alkaloids in commercial comfrey products." *Journal of Pharmaceutical Sciences* 83 (5): 649–53.

Bove, M. 1996. *An Encyclopedia of Natural Healing for Children and Infants*. Los Angeles: Keats Publishing.

Brooke, E. 1992. *A Woman's Book of Herbs*. London: The Women's Press.

de Vries, J. 1995. *Pregnancy and Childbirth*. Edinburgh: Mainstream Publishing.

Fenwick, E. 1996. *101 Essential Tips for Baby Care*. New York: Dorling Kindersley.

Gladstar, R. 1993. *Herbal Healing for Women*. New York: Simon & Schuster.

Hudson, T. 1999. *Women's Encyclopedia of Natural Medicine*. Los Angeles: Keats Publishing.

Jordan, Sandra. 1988. *Yoga for Pregnancy: Safe and Gentle Stretches*. New York: St. Martin's Press.

Lincoln, D. 1994. Report of the director of the Medical Research Council's Reproductive Biology Unit to the British Association for the Advancement of Science meeting, September.

McIntyre, A. 1988. *Herbs for Pregnancy and Childbirth*. London: Sheldon Press.

———. 1994. *The Complete Woman's Herbal*. London: Gaia Books.

Ody, P. 1995. *Home Herbal*. New York: Dorling Kindersley.

Parvati, J. 1979. *Hygieia: A Woman's Herbal.* London: Wildwood House.

Rogers, C. 1995. *The Women's Guide to Herbal Medicine.* London: Hamish Hamilton.

Schouenborg, L. O. et al. 1992. "Hyperemesis gravidarum." *Ugeski-Laeger* 154: 1015–19.

Weed, S. 1986. *Wise Woman Herbal for the Childbearing Year.* Woodstock, N.Y.: Ash Tree Publishing.

Index

A

abdominal pain, 23–24

afterpains, 62

agrimony, 44, 68, 77, 148
   actions/uses, 92

alcohol consumption, 2, 4, 17, 45

alder buckthorn, caution, 86

allergies, 24–25

aloe
   actions/uses, 92–93
   caution, 81, 93

aluminum, 3

American ginseng, 33
   actions/uses, 93

amniotic fluid, release of, 55

anemia, iron-deficiency, 17–18, 25–27, 33

angelica, caution, 86

anise, 35, 68
   actions/uses, 93–94
   caution, 86

antioxidants, 4

arbor vitae, caution, 81

arnica
   actions/uses, 94
   caution, 94

arnica 6X, 48, 56, 59

aromatherapy oils, 145

autumn crocus, caution, 81

B

babies
   breast-feeding, 67–71
   colds, 73–74
   colic, 74–75
   cradle cap, 75
   diaper rash, 76
   eye problems, 76–77
   herbal teas for, 74–75
   jaundiced, 77

massaging, 22
sleepless, 78–79
teething, 79
umbilical cord care, 79–80
uniqueness of, 73
yeast infections, 71, 80

Bach Flower Remedies, 41, 42, 49, 56, 57, 64, 66, 152
Rescue Remedy, 32–33, 48, 65
suggested uses, 42

backache, 27–28

bacteria in foods, 4–5, 17

barberry
caution, 81

basil, 56, 58, 64
actions/uses, 94–95
caution, 81, 95

baths, 27–28, 37, 41, 49, 51

bed rest, 51, 52

beta-carotene, 3–4

beth root, 54
actions/uses, 95
caution, 81, 95

bistort, 44
actions/uses, 95–96

bitter orange, 39
actions/uses, 96
caution, 86

black cohosh, 54, 56, 57, 62
actions/uses, 96–97
caution, 82

black haw, 24, 29, 52, 56, 62
actions/uses, 97

black horehound, 39, 54
actions/uses, 97

bladder problems, 28

bleeding, herbs for, 52

blessed thistle, 54
actions/uses, 98
caution, 98

blood pressure
high, 48–49
low, 32–33
normal range, in pregnancy, 48

blood pressure checks, 47

bloodroot, caution, 82

blue cohosh, 54, 57
caution, 82

bonding, 67

borage, 63, 70
actions/uses, 99–100
caution, 100

Braxton Hicks contractions, 24

breast engorgement, 69

breast-feeding, 25, 62, 65, 67–71
herbal teas for, 68
preparing for, 67–69
supplementing, 70

breast milk, 67
  advantages of, 67
  insufficient, 69–70
  jaundice in babies and, 77

breathing exercises, 19–20, 29, 41

breathlessness, 29

breech babies, 54–55

broom, caution, 82

bugleweed, caution, 82

burdock, 27
  actions/uses, 100

butternut
  actions/uses, 100

buying herbs, 148

C

cabbage leaves, 70

caffeine, 5, 17, 27, 49, 79, 90

calcium, 25, 27, 37, 38, 44

Californian Flower Quintessentials, 34, 41
  suggested uses, 43

caloric needs, 14–15

camphor
  actions/uses, 101
  caution, 101

Candida albicans, 44

candidiasis, 5, 71

caraway, 68, 70, 75
  actions/uses, 101
  caution, 86, 102

carpel tunnel syndrome, 29–30

carrot juice, 36

cascara sagrada, caution, 86

catmint, 34, 74, 78
  actions/uses, 102

celery seed, caution, 86

chamomile, 25, 28, 29, 33, 34, 36, 37, 39, 40, 41, 45, 56, 64, 69, 71, 74, 75, 78, 79
  actions/uses, 102–103
  caution, 86

Chamomilla 3X, 75, 79, 103

chaste tree, 7, 48, 70
  actions/uses, 103
  caution, 103

childbirth. *See also* labor
  herbal support for, 53–54, 56, 57, 58
  planning for, 1–7

chili, caution, 86

Chinese foxglove, 52

Chinese traditional medicine, 1–2, 39, 52, 65–66, 75, 78, 79 cinnamon, caution, 87

cleavers, 32
   actions/uses, 103–104

cloves
   actions/uses, 104
   caution, 82, 104

coffee. *See* caffeine

colds, baby's, 73–74

colic, 74–75

colostrum, 67

comfrey, 63, 76
   actions/uses, 104
   caution, 82, 105

compresses
   cold, 35, 36, 145
   preparing, 146
   warm, 37–38, 57, 69, 146

conception, 6. *See also* preconceptual period

conjunctivitis, in babies, 76

constipation, 12
   causes of, 30

contractions
   of labor, 55, 57–58
   prelabor, 55

cornsilk, 28, 32
   actions/uses, 105–106

cotton root, caution, 82

couch grass, 28, 32
   actions/uses, 105

cowslip, caution, 87

cradle cap, 75–76

cramp bark, 24, 29, 38
   actions/uses, 106

cranberry, 28
   actions/uses, 106–107

cravings, and anemia, 17–18

creativity during pregnancy, 34

Culpepper, Nicholas, xv

cystitis, 5, 28

D

damiana, 6, 41, 65
   actions/uses, 107

dandelion, 27, 32, 77
   actions/uses, 107–108

decoctions, preparing, 144

depression, postnatal, 63–64

devil's claw, caution, 82

diaper rash, 76

diet during pregnancy, 14–18, 33

digestive tract, 12

dill, 68, 70, 75
   actions/uses, 108

discomforts of pregnancy, herbs for, 23–46

diuretics, herbal, 31–32

dong quai, 7, 52, 65–66
    actions/uses, 108
    caution, 7, 83, 109

E

echinacea, 7, 28, 73, 79–80
    actions/uses, 109

ectopic pregnancy, 47–50

edema (fluid retention), 31–32

elder, 40, 45, 74
    actions/uses, 109–110
    caution, 87

embryonic development, 9

emotional disturbances. *See also* stress
    herbs for, 33–34
    sinusitis and, 40

emotional problems, 12–13

endometriosis, 5

energy, Traditional Chinese Medicine on, 1–2

episiotomy, avoidance of, 58

essential oils, 74, 145, 148

eucalyptus, 74

exercise, 18–20, 29, 30

eye problems, baby's, 76–77

F

fainting, causes of, 32

false labor pains, 24

false unicorn root (helonias), 7, 39, 52, 54
    actions/uses, 110
    caution, 83, 110

fatigue, 33–34
    after childbirth, 64, 65
    morning sickness and, 38–39

fennel, 35, 39, 40, 68, 70, 75
    actions/uses, 110–111
    caution, 87

fenugreek, 70
    actions/uses, 111
    caution, 87, 111

fertility, female, 5–7

fertility, male, 2–3, 6

fertilization techniques, 5

fetal abnormalities, 9

fetal development, monthly progress, 9–10

feverfew, caution, 83

fiber in diet, 30

fluid loss, 38–39

fluid retention, 31–32, 45

folic acid, 3–4, 26

food additives, 2, 4

foods
    to avoid during pregnancy, 4–5, 16–17
    cravings, 17

iron-rich, 18

G

garlic, 7, 33
    actions/uses, 111–112
    caution, 87, 112

ginger, 38–39, 40, 56, 62
    actions/uses, 112

ginseng (*Panax ginseng*), 6, 33
    actions/uses, 113
    caution, 33, 87

glossary, 151–155

goat's rue, 70
    actions/uses, 113
    caution, 113

golden seal, caution, 83

gotu kola, caution, 87

greater celandine, caution, 83

grief after loss of newborn, 66

gum problems, 44

H

hawthorn, 27, 33, 38, 49
    actions/uses, 114

hay fever, 24

heartburn, 34–35

heartsease, 75, 76
    actions/uses, 114

helonias. *See* false unicorn root

hemorrhoids, treatment of, 35

herbs
    to avoid completely during pregnancy, 4, 17, 30, 33, 81–85, 92
    buying and storing, 148
    organic, 148
    preparation of, 143–148
    suppliers, 149
    top ten for childbirth/postnatal period, 91
    top ten for pregnancy use, 91
    to use in moderation during pregnancy, 86–90

hiatal hernia, 36

hormone regulators, herbal, 48

horse chestnut, 46
    actions/uses, 115

horsetail, 32
    actions/uses, 114–115

hospital confinement, 61

hypertension, 48–49

I

immune system, baby's, 73

infertility. *See* fertility

infusions, preparing, 143–144

insomnia. *See* sleeplessness

iron in diet, 17–18, 26

ispaghula. *See* psyllium

J

jasmine
  actions/uses, 116
  caution, 87

jaundice, in babies, 77

Jiao Ai Tang, 52

jing, 1, 2

Jordan, Sandra, 18

juniper, caution, 83

K

kelp, 27
  actions/uses, 116–117
  caution, 117

Korean ginseng. *See* ginseng (*Panax ginseng*)

L

labor. *See also* childbirth
  encouraging, 55
  stages of, 55, 57–59

lady's mantle, 6, 44, 48, 54
  actions/uses, 117
  caution, 83, 117

lavender, 24, 63, 69, 70, 74
  actions/uses, 117–118
  caution, 88

laxatives, herbal, 35
  caution, 30–31

lead, 3

leg cramps, 37–38

lemon, actions/uses, 118

lemon balm, 33, 34, 39, 41, 63, 64, 78
  actions/uses, 118–119

licorice
  actions/uses, 119
  caution, 119

licorice, caution, 88

liferoot, caution, 83

lifestyle, 6

lime flowers, 33, 41, 49, 79
  actions/uses, 119–120

lovage, caution, 88

M

magnesium, 27

marigold, 6, 25, 44–45, 56, 57, 63, 69, 71, 75, 76
  actions/uses, 120

marjoram, caution, 88

marshmallow, 35
  actions/uses, 120–121

massage, 21–22, 24, 38, 42–43, 56, 57
  for breech baby, 55
  for calming babies, 76
  for carpel tunnel syndrome, 29
  for colic in babies, 75
  for edema, 32

massage oils, 145–146

mastitis, 69, 70–71

materia medica, 91–141

meadowsweet, 35, 36, 50
   actions/uses, 121
   caution, 121

medical check, six-week, 61

medications, unnecessary, avoiding, 4, 7, 17

melilot, 46
   actions/uses, 122
   caution, 122

midwives, xv–xvi, 21, 54, 67–68

milk thistle, 70
   actions/uses, 122
   caution, 122

minerals, dietary sources, 16

miscarriage, 9
   threatened, 51–52

mistletoe, caution, 83

morning sickness, 38–40

motherwort, 24, 54, 56, 57, 58
   actions/uses, 122–123
   caution, 88, 123

mugwort, 52, 56, 57
   actions/uses, 123
   caution, 83, 123

myrrh, caution, 88

N

nasal congestion, 74

neroli, actions/uses, 123–124

nervines, 64

nipples, 67, 69, 71

nutmeg
   actions/uses, 124
   caution, 88, 124

O

oak, actions/uses, 124–125

oats, 41
   actions/uses, 125

oils, 42–43, 57, 70
   infused, hot and cold, preparing, 145
   massage, 145–146

oregano, caution, 88

ovarian cysts, 5

oxytocin, 55

P

pain, abdominal, 23–24

parenthood, shock of, 64–65

parsley
   actions/uses, 125–125
   caution, 88, 126

partus praeparators, 53–54

passion flower, 29, 37, 49
   actions/uses, 126

caution, 89

patchouli, actions/uses, 126

pennyroyal, caution, 84

pepper, black, actions/uses, 98

peppermint, 6–7, 39–40
  actions/uses, 127
  caution, 89, 127

perineum problems, 62–63

Peruvian bark, caution, 84

pesticides, 2–3

pilewort, 35, 63
  actions/uses, 127–128

placenta, 10
  expulsion of, 58

plaintain, 70
  actions/uses, 128

pokeroot, caution, 84

pollution, 2–3, 4

postnatal care, 61–71

posture, 20, 27

potassium, 33, 50

poultices, preparing, 146

preconceptual period, 2–5

preeclampsia, 48, 49–50

pregnancy
  diagnosis of, 11
  ectopic, 47–50
  fetus's monthly progress, 9–10
  hormonal changes during, 12
  mother's monthly progress, 11–13
  second trimester, 12

prostaglandins, 55

protein needs, 15

psyllium/ispaghula, 30, 35
  actions/uses, 115–116
  caution, 116

pulsatilla, caution, 84

Q

qi, 1–2, 39, 154

qigong, 19, 20

R

raspberry leaf, 53, 54, 56, 57, 58, 62, 65
  actions/uses, 128
  caution, 89, 129

red clover, 6, 71
  actions/uses, 129

relaxation, 41

Rescue Remedy. *See under* Bach Flower Remedies

rhubarb root, caution, 8 9

rose, actions/uses, 129–130

rose geranium oil, actions/uses, 130

rosehips, 27

rosemary, 65, 79
    actions/uses, 130–131
    caution, 89, 131

rue, caution, 84

S

saffron, caution, 89

sage, 48, 56, 57, 66, 79
    actions/uses, 131
    caution, 89

St. John's wort, 28, 37, 54, 56, 63–64
    actions/uses, 135–136
    caution, 136

salt intake, 16–17

sandalwood, actions/uses, 131–132

sassafras, caution, 84

saw palmetto, 6, 70
    actions/uses, 132

senna, 30
    caution, 89

sesame, actions/uses, 133

sexual intercourse
    during labor, 55
    during pregnancy, 13–14

shepherd's purse, 46, 58
    actions/uses, 132–133
    caution, 84

"show," 55

Siberian ginseng, 33, 41
    actions/uses, 133

sinusitis, 40

skin rashes, 25

skullcap, 27, 33, 37, 41
    actions/uses, 134

sleeplessness, 12, 36–37, 65

slippery elm, 35, 36, 40
    actions/uses, 134

smoking, 2, 3

southernwood, caution, 84

spearmint, 35, 74
    actions/uses, 135

squatting, 20

squaw vine, 54, 62
    actions/uses, 135

squill, caution, 85

stillbirth, 66

stinging nettle, 6, 26–27, 38, 70
    action/uses, 136

storing herbs, 148

stress, 34, 41–42
    Bach Flower Remedies for, 41, 42, 49
    Californian Flower Quintessentials for, 41

    conception and, 6
    herbs for, 41
    hypertension and, 49
    shock of parenthood, 64–65

stretch marks, 42–44

sugar, 45

suppliers of herbs, 149

swimming, 19

symphysis pubis dysfunction (SPD), 50–51

T

tansy, caution, 85

teas, caffeine-containing, 5, 90
  caution, 90

teas, herbal
  for babies, 74–75
  combined infusions and decoctions, 144
  decoctions, 144
  infusions, 143–144

tea tree oil, 74, 76
  actions/uses, 137

teeth and gum problems, 44

teething, 79

thyme, caution, 90

Tierra, Michael, xvi

tinctures
  alcohol in, 146, 147, 155
  diluted, 39
  preparing, 147–148

toxoplasmosis, 17

U

umbilical cord care, 79–80

urinary tract infections, 28

urine checks, 47

uterine contraction after birth, 62

uva-ursi, 28, 50
  actions/uses, 137

V

vaginal yeast infection, 44–45

varicose veins, 45–46

vegetarian diet, 15, 26, 49

vervain, 63, 70, 74
  actions/uses, 137–138
  caution, 90, 138

vitamin A, 17, 26

vitamin B6 XX sub, 29–30

vitamin C, 18

vitamins, 3–4
  dietary sources, 16

W

water, bottled, 4

watercress, actions/uses, 138

water systems, 2–3, 4

Weed, Susun, 1

weight gain, 14, 15

white horehound, caution, 90

white willow, 50
  actions/uses, 138–139
  caution, 139

wild yam, 57, 62
  actions/uses, 139
  caution, 85, 139

winter cherry, 6
  actions/uses, 139–140

Wise Woman Herbal for the Childbearing Year (Weed), 1

witch hazel, 35, 45–4 6, 63
  actions/uses, 140

wood betony, 56, 57, 78
  actions/uses, 140
  caution, 90, 141

work, 64

wormwood, caution, 85

Y

yarrow, caution, 90

yeast infections
  in babies, 71, 76, 80
  vaginal, 44–45

yellow dock, 31
  actions/uses, 141

yoga, 18–19, 20, 27

Yoga for Pregnancy (Jordan), 18

Z

zinc, 4

Meera.
~~Megan~~
Nayan
Mischa.
Nikita
Joshua
Luke